LEAVE

A POSTPARTUM ACCOUNT

Shayne Terry

Autofocus Books
Easton, PA | Orlando, FL

Published by Autofocus Books
autofocusbooks.com

1st printing

Essay/Literature
ISBN: 978-1-957392-35-6

Library of Congress Control Number: 2024944057

LEAVE

A POSTPARTUM ACCOUNT

For my mother

BIRTH STORIES, PART I

There are several versions of the birth story.

There is the short, light version. "The labor was quick—so quick that we almost didn't make it to the hospital." The baby is healthy. The baby is beautiful. We love the baby. Words that are true but that hide other truths.

Then there is the long, comic version that Daniel and I tell together, playing off each other. The unruly contractions, the quick transition. Speeding to the hospital in a thunderstorm, me on my knees in the backseat, breathing to hold in the baby—"the longest car ride of my life!" Stomping through puddles and pouring rain in my bare feet because there was no time for shoes and bypassing triage altogether after being measured at 10 centimeters plus two. The doctor rushing in and asking, "Why isn't this patient's information on the screen?" A nurse replying, "We don't even know her name."

There is the brief version that hints at trouble. The baby came shooting out. Tore right out of there. Ripped his way into the world. I lead with this when I don't know how much a person wants to know, how much they can take, how responsible a listener they will be. Not everyone can be trusted with pain. Not everyone can hold someone else's pain along with their own.

With most of my friends, I stick to the basic facts: I tore badly. It hurts more than I imagined, and in different ways. The recovery will be long.

STITCHED, PART I

At first, I am relieved that it's over so quickly. The baby is placed on my chest, where he pees on me, another warm liquid to mingle with the blood and the rain and the amniotic fluid, and then inches his way toward my nipple to feed. It is just like the video we saw in our birth class, that first human instinct on show.

I barely notice the placenta being delivered, the medical staff buzzing around my feet, until the doctor looks up from between my legs and says, "I'm sorry. There was no way to prevent it." She tells me she will need to do some stitching.

I expected a few stitches. I smile. I look at my baby, who is falling into his first sleep in this world. I look at Daniel, so proud. I am not worried about a few stitches.

The doctor is down there for a long time. Occasionally she calls to the nurse to bring her more anesthetic. Another nurse takes the baby across the room to be examined, then down the hall for some tests. Someone gives me a hospital ID bracelet and brings me consent forms to sign, saying it is okay for them to deliver my baby. We laugh about how backward it all is.

Then the stitching becomes more uncomfortable. The

soreness starts to set in. After an hour, I ask, "How many stitches am I getting?"

With a forced brightness, the doctor says, "We prefer to think of it as one big suture."

I wait a while and ask again, but she only changes the subject. I never get a straight answer, but when, after a few weeks, I finally get up the courage to hold a mirror to myself, all I see is black embroidery.

PAIN

When I was young, my family called my grandmother The Pharmacy. Entire drawers in her kitchen and bathroom were full of orange pill bottles, labels with her name and dosage guidelines that she ignored. Loose capsules filled the space between bottles, but she always seemed to know what each one did.

She was a med pusher like some grandmas are food pushers. "You look tired," she'd say. "I have something for that." Into your hand she'd drop a large white pill, a small pink one. If you said you had a headache, felt congested, had sore muscles, she had something for that. "You seem depressed," she would say. "Take this." Prozac, Percocet, Vicodin, Valium. I don't remember seeing my grandmother eat much, but I have a clear picture of her tossing a pill to the back of her throat and downing it with Diet Pepsi. I can see her rummaging through her drawers to find the perfect prescription for one of my uncles, for my mother, for me. This was what a grandmother was: someone who could stop pain.

At some point, the adults became uneasy about it and stopped calling her The Pharmacy. It stopped being funny when she had to go to rehab for her codeine addiction, when she had to go back because she overdosed again.

I was in high school the first time my mother and her brothers looted my grandmother's house and trashed all her prescriptions, when they began the long battle with her doctors to figure out who was acting as her dispensary. I remember my mother's defeat when she realized that while each doctor was arguably overprescribing to some degree, my grandmother was playing a more sophisticated game. She had a whole army of doctors at different health systems and hospitals, each of whom thought they were the only one. She knew what symptoms to play up to get the pills she wanted, what not to say to avoid sounding alarms. She had mail-order drugs with automatic refills. Every time her drawers and cabinets were cleaned out, she managed to fill them back up.

It's not that she isn't in pain. She is, and has been my whole life—migraines, stomach problems, arthritis, constant trouble with her uterus that led to a hysterectomy—but it's difficult to know how much of her pain is primary, and how much is caused by her homemade drug concoctions. Her chief complaint is headaches, followed by dizziness. In recent years, she has medicated herself to the point that she can't walk without support. Sometimes when I call she is coherent, but often she slurs her words or says them out of order. More often, she is sleeping. Once, I asked her why she takes the pills that make her drowsy, and she said, "I'd rather be asleep than awake."

It is two in the morning. My baby is four hours old, and I have finally been moved from the delivery room to a shared room in the Mother and Baby unit. Two nurses stand over my bed: the kind one who helped deliver my baby and talked to me through the stitching, and the one who will be taking care of me on this new floor.

"She doesn't want the pain meds," the kind nurse says to the new one.

"Why not?" The new nurse turns to me. "Why not?" I can't explain my grandmother, how the drugs turn her into someone else. Instead I say, "I just had a baby without anything. I don't want to start now."

The kind nurse tells me that the drugs will simply help me get some sleep. I don't want to risk constipation, I say. The new nurse says, just take one pill, one pill won't hurt.

It is then that I realize the whiteboard at the end of my bed, the one that says "Pain Management: Percocet," is not left over from another patient but has been written up for me. I feel so tired.

The new nurse leans over my bed, stern. "You won't be able to take care of your baby if you're in pain."

I look at the baby, sleeping in a clear plastic bassinet next to my hospital bed. "Okay."

Back to the birth story: it didn't actually happen that fast.

I had heard all the stories about first births, how they take forever, and I'd mentally prepared myself for 24, 36, 48 hours of labor, a slow buildup to a drawn-out finale. From start to finish, mine was 16 hours.

I woke up in early labor. I notified our doula and then passed the morning going on leisurely walks and paying medical bills.

Over the course of the day, my contractions grew stronger. I withstood the waves of discomfort by leaning forward and pushing against the kitchen counter. Daniel timed each one and we waited for the contractions to regulate and get closer together, as we'd been told by all the birth books they would, but they were all over the place: a 30-second contraction followed by a seven-minute break, a one-minute contraction followed by a 20-minute break, two 45-second contractions with barely any break at all. I felt them in my back rather than my belly. I called the doula again in the afternoon, and she told me we still had a ways to go, that we should hunker down for the night, to call when I thought I needed her.

By early evening, I was vomiting between contractions. I tried to rate my pain, but I wasn't sure. Was this a five out of ten? An eight out of ten? Was the intensity to come beyond my imagination of pain?

Some people have the worldview that all pain should be treated, prevented, eradicated. If it is possible to be without pain, why suffer? Then there is the opposing viewpoint: pain is our body's way of communicating that something is wrong; mask it and we miss the message. These are extremes; most people live somewhere in the middle. But I find that difficult.

After witnessing my grandmother's gradual addiction to pain pills, I developed a strong aversion to even over-the-counter medications. I shouldered my way through sinus infections, stitches, broken bones and was lucky, for more than a decade, to experience no pain I couldn't handle. I began to say that I had a high pain tolerance, but the truth was that the pain I encountered was more tolerable to me than what I perceived to be the known and unknown risks of drugs.

When, in my early thirties, my period cramps became more intense and my friends suggested ibuprofen, the concept of "taking something" had become so foreign that it hadn't even occurred to me as a possibility. I was amazed when I tried it and it worked.

Around that time, one of those friends shared that her mother had asked her if she knew anyone affected by the opioid epidemic. Laughing, she said she told her mother she didn't hang around people like that. I pictured my grandmother: frail, shaky.

Neither I nor my friend had ever experienced chronic pain. For those who haven't lived in chronic pain or watched a loved one live through it, it can be easy to judge. My grandmother's need for something to dull the pain in her life has always been real. It doesn't matter where that pain comes from. The profundity of pain is that it has both physical and emotional components, and one can feed off—or starve—the other.

The Percocet does not help me sleep, because my roommate's baby wails all night. Her baby is having trouble latching, and the woman repeatedly asks the nurses for a spoon so that she can express by hand and satisfy its hunger. At six, the same nurse who insisted I deal with my pain so that I could take care of my baby comes in and scolds my roommate. "It's a baby. It's crying because it needs something. You can't just let it cry." No one ever brings a spoon.

I stand my ground. I don't want any more Percocet, but I accept the ibuprofen offered by the nurses every six hours. I begin to feel my pain, and my pain scares me. The injury runs right through the core of me, front to back, rendering me immobile. I can't shift my position in the bed, let alone make it to the bathroom without Daniel practically carrying me there, supporting me while I pee. In my memory of those bathroom trips, tears stream down my face, but I may have been too shocked to cry.

Pain does not have to mean suffering, according to the compact, energetic woman who taught our birth class. Pain that has a purpose, like the purpose of bringing your baby into this world, can be the fact of pain without the feeling of suffering. I went into labor with no fear. It was painful, yes, but the woman was right; I did not suffer. Not until after the birth.

THE FIELD

A few days after the birth, I consider what would have happened to me without medical care. The likelihood of my death seems high, if not from the tearing and the loss of blood, then from an infection.

I imagine myself a hundred years ago, when the maternal mortality ratio in the U.S. was 36 times higher and puerperal fever—a blanket term for the postpartum bacterial infections that regularly swept maternity wards, transmitted from one doctor to multiple patients—could easily lead to sepsis and death.

Or today, in Sub-Saharan Africa, where the majority of this century's maternal deaths have occurred; in Sierra Leone, around 1 in 75 pregnancies ends in the death of the mother.

Or today, in the U.S. as a Black or Indigenous woman, who, at my age and with my same level of education, is 5.2 times more likely to die from pregnancy-related causes than I am as a white woman.

By now, we know the numbers. ("Well, we should," my friend Rachel says.) But each one of those labors began with a contraction. Perhaps her contractions were unruly, perhaps her transition was quick. Perhaps before her death she endured the longest car ride of her life.

I lived, and I should feel grateful, but I don't. I feel like I am standing in the doorway of a house, looking out onto a field strewn with bodies. It is the aftermath of some battle in a war as old as us, the bodies of all the women who never made it to this threshold.

But birth is not a war. Birth happens during war, birth happens despite war, birth is made more dangerous by war.

I want to turn, to go inside the house, but the house is dark and there is no one to beckon me in, so I stand here in the doorway, alone.

BABY CARE

For the first five weeks, I do not care for the baby at all. I lie on the couch, barely able to turn my body from one side to the other. Even small, slow movements produce the kind of pain that is a warning sign to stop before something else breaks. When I must stand, I get lightheaded and dizzy, and I have to use the wall as support just to make it to the bathroom.

At night, baby care falls on Daniel. He changes all the diapers and tracks the pees and poops and feedings in a log at which I do not look.

During the day, there is a carousel of women: my mother, my mother-in-law, my sister, my mother again. They each stay for a week, sleeping on an air mattress on our living room floor. They dress the baby and hold him and change him and talk to him. They bring him to me on the couch and lay him next to me so he can feed. He latches on his own and I read on my phone, often forgetting he is there. All I want is a book good enough to help me forget my body for a while. My only goal each day is to get to the next because I have been promised that eventually all the days will add up to less pain.

AN ABRIDGED SEARCH HISTORY, PART I

how to care for third degree tear
postpartum fluid leakage
is it okay to fall asleep while breastfeeding
can you use colace and miralax together
postpartum stitches bleeding
postpartum stitches when to call doctor
does eating make constipation worse
how much bleeding is normal after birth
when do babies start seeing color
sharp abdominal pain 2 weeks postpartum
high waisted underwear
best diaper rash cream
talc baby powder lawsuit
how to stream democratic debate
how to revive fiddle leaf fig dying
how to burp sleeping baby
sitz bath doesn't fit on toilet
sitz bath puts pressure on hemorrhoids
severe pain after third degree tear

NORMAL

It's hard to know whether my pain is normal, because women don't usually go public with their postpartum symptoms. I have never personally heard anyone talk about going through what I am going through, although neither am I talking explicitly about it—not to the family members who are caring for me, not to Daniel, and barely to my doctor. It's not that I don't want to talk about it; rather, I don't have the precise language to locate the pain.

I obsessively search online. I find the clinical term: obstetric anal sphincter injuries (OASIS, ironically) are tears that go beyond the perineum and into the anal sphincter. These tears are classified as either third- or fourth-degree. Both degrees involve a tear of the muscle that surrounds the anus, but fourth-degree tears extend into the rectal mucosa.

I read the long list of symptoms and complications and then wish I hadn't. Most common: pelvic pain, urinary incontinence, and anal incontinence, meaning uncontrollable bowels and leakage of feces. Also possible: a prolapse, when an organ such as the bladder slips down from its normal position and bulges into the vagina, or a fistula, an opening between the vagina and either the bladder or the rectum. Dyspareunia—pain during intercourse—is not unusual.

I keep searching.

oasis what are the chances

But the medical literature is all over the place. One article says OASIS occur in .1% of vaginal births, while the next article says it could be up to 11%. Researchers seem to agree that rates vary by country and have been rising over the last several decades—possibly due to improved diagnostics, though there are other theories, mainly that first-time moms are getting older and heavier.

Some days, perversely, I wish that the injury were more prevalent than it seems, that though it's rarely spoken of, there are plenty of other women who have been here. That I am less alone than I feel.

LEAVE, PART I

I have ten weeks of paid leave, provided by New York's Paid Family Leave law. The new law is still rolling out and will eventually mandate twelve, but ten weeks of paid leave is better than what I am offered by the company where I work, which is zero.

My mother started the company, a marketing agency, when I was eight. This was after she got her MBA, going to school at night while working full-time with two little kids at home. I always swore I'd never go into the family business, but around the time I turned thirty I stopped seeing the company as my competition for her attention and began to understand it as something she made, partially for me. I joined and grew to love the quirky little agency she built, but working for my mother comes with its complications.

One of the first things my mother said when she found out I was pregnant was, "You know you don't have maternity leave."

I informed her that, although our company is based in Illinois, New York's new law covered me, as a remote employee paying taxes here. I expected her to be pleased, but she seemed almost annoyed. Was she disappointed that I wouldn't be forced to do what she did after her babies, run out my PTO and get back to work?

My mother is one of those women who refuses to call herself a feminist because she believes hard work is all that got her where she is, and it would have been hard work for a woman or a man. She will insist that she was never discriminated against in the same breath that she tells you about the male boss she got fired for sexually harassing her. ("I didn't get him fired," she says. "He got himself fired.")

As my mother, she was thrilled that I was having a baby. As a small business owner, there were other factors to consider. As a woman… but my mother would never begin a sentence that way.

Given my situation, I was happy with the ten weeks provided by the state.

But it is already apparent that my leave will not look anything like I had imagined. Two weeks in—twenty percent of my leave, gone—I have not yet been able to stand up straight. My body is a hinge that rusted halfway closed. I have not walked, aside from trips to the bathroom and two excruciating, exhausting doctor visits, one for the baby and one for me. Because my stitches are so extensive, the doctor wants to see me sooner than the usual six-week follow-up, and though getting from our apartment to the car and from the car to her office seems nearly impossible, I am thankful for the validation that

I am not crazy, that this is not normal.

Leaning on Daniel for support, I pause to look at myself in the mirror in our building lobby. My skin is a sickly pale yellow, a bruise-colored half-moon beneath each eye. Bent, hobbled, I look like an old woman. I look like my grandmother.

HOLDING, PART I

My grandmother calls often to check on me after the birth. Of the handful of people who know what happened to me, she has the most genuine empathy for my pain. I can hear it in her voice, how she is allowing herself to break with sadness for me.

She had five children in quick succession, the first when she was eighteen. Her first husband was abusive, and only now do I realize what that must have meant for her in the aftermath of childbirth.

"I had a friend," she tells me, "who would come over every night and sit with me and hold the baby while I took a bath."

I imagine this other woman, perched on the toilet in a cramped, butter-yellow bathroom, cradling my newborn uncle while my grandmother lay naked in the clear, hot water. I can feel my grandmother willing the water to heal her. I can feel how much it hurts to step in and out of the tub, can see my grandmother's friend offering a strong arm for support. Holding her baby and holding her.

"She was a good friend," my grandmother says.

I tell my mother, the first in the line-up of visiting caretakers, about my grandmother's friend who sat with her and held her baby while she bathed.

"That would be Tootsie," my mother says. "They were best friends."

She tells me that there was a group of young mothers who all lived on the same street. My grandmother, Tootsie, Charmaine, and Lillian. They helped each other, she says, implying that they got no help from their husbands or, for women like my grandmother, from their mothers.

I have never known my grandmother to have a best friend or even a close friend. "What a loss," I say. "When did Tootsie die?"

"Oh, Tootsie's alive," my mother says. "I asked if I could invite her to the birthday party." My grandmother is turning eighty at the of the summer. "But Grandma said no."

"Why?"

My mother gives me a look that says she has tried. "I think she doesn't want anyone to see her like this."

SHITTY THINGS

One by one, close friends come to visit. They sit in the chair and I lie on the couch, which is actually a loveseat, and which has begun to smell sour from the breast milk that has dribbled from the baby's mouth and soaked into the cushions, leaving white stains on the dark gray wool.

I am mostly honest about how terrible things are, to different degrees.

I have three friends who are pregnant, and with them I am cagey. On the one hand, I wish I had known about the possibility of a birth injury. On the other hand, the chances that they will go through what I am going through are slim. To tell them would scare them, likely needlessly. I still believe that it is better to go into birth without fear, even though there is plenty to be afraid of. Knowing about everything that can go wrong during birth is helpful if one is deciding whether or not to have a baby, I reason. Once one has made the decision, fear has no utility. I skate over the details with my pregnant friends. No, I can't walk yet. Yes, I tore, but I am healing. Yes, I have had some setbacks, but overall—progress.

I cannot bring myself to speak candidly to my friend who had cancer. She is not even a year in remission. She comes to sit with me, an echo of the summer before, when our small circle of friends would accompany her to chemo. She lost her hair, she lost weight, and for a while she lost her ability to run, a thing she loved to do and was very good at.

When she comes to visit me, she is still in the process of recovering her life. Her hair is short and spunky, a style that her pre-cancer self never would have chosen but that looks good on her. She is wearing a dress with a cutout that reveals her back, also something I can't picture her wearing before she got sick and got better. She sits across from my mother-in-law, that week's designated caretaker, and I do my best to prop myself up in a near-sitting position, a long side lean that, while it uses energy I do not have, doesn't put pressure on the parts of me that hurt.

Being honest with this friend feels like complaining. She had it so much worse, I think. The unknowns that come with cancer—where the disease came from, whether it's spreading at any given moment—are objectively scarier than an injury whose origins can be traced and, to some extent, explained. And while my life would have been in danger had I not had proper medical care, she faced a disease that is still in large part a mystery to us, something that might have easily resulted in her death despite the doctors doing their best.

I also know that, before starting chemo and radiation, my friend froze her eggs, because the treatment for the cancer was risky to her reproductive system. I know that she wanted a baby, probably still wants one. I don't know how long she has been advised to wait before trying. I don't know if she has been trying already.

My situation seems almost silly compared to what my friend has gone through, and I tell her this. "It's nothing compared to cancer."

"But it still blows," she says. "We all have our shitty things, and just because they're different doesn't mean one is less shitty than the other."

It's a relief to hear her say this, as if she has given me permission to be sad about what happened to me.

"Yes," I say. "It really blows."

BLAME

In the weeks after the birth, I look for someone to blame. The doctor, for telling me it was okay to push. Our doula, for not coming sooner, for not knowing that I was in active labor when we spoke on the phone. Myself, for not doing enough perineal massage during the third trimester. Most of the blame I put on myself.

What if we had gone to the hospital sooner? What if I'd had a midwife instead of an obstetrician? What if I had rested more during my third trimester? What if I had read just one more book about labor?

I search again.

can a third degree tear be prevented

I expect to receive a litany of the things I did wrong, or didn't do and should have. Instead, I see the same result, repeated over and over by medical journals in articles and meta-analyses: third- and fourth-degree tears cannot be prevented because they cannot be anticipated. Trying to prevent them by increasing the cesarean section rate would require that a large number of cesarean sections be done to prevent a small number of tears.

I feel almost disappointed that there is no one to blame.

In a way, it would be easier if there were. Instead, I am left with free-floating anger and sadness and nowhere to direct it, not even at myself.

WHY

As our due dates approached, my pregnant friends were like corn kernels in hot oil, all wondering who would pop next. Each new explosion set off a text chain of news. How was baby? How was mom? How long was the labor?

Those who went before me seemed to have relatively easy births. I wonder now if they just said that. One kernel to another: it doesn't hurt that bad.

They seem to be experiencing straightforward recoveries: I witness them walking around, holding their babies, turning to say hello with no sign of the excruciating pain that I am now experiencing with the smallest of movements.

Unfair is not the right word for it. There are no judicial scales when it comes to the pain we are dealt in life. My question is not why me; it is simply why.

I remember the host of a podcast I once listened to referring to her "traumatic birth story," a phrase that meant nothing to me at the time and now is so heavy with meaning I feel it in the bones around my heart, like a damper pedal on my lungs. I look her up and find the episode in which she tells her story in full and interviews her midwife in an attempt to process what happened to her.

At first, I am terrified. This woman is several years out from her birth, but the emotional pain of it is clearly tender, an exposed wire on the surface of her life. Will that be me, five years from now? I recognize my current situation in her story: unable to walk or climb stairs, unable to hold or carry the baby, unable to stand long enough to change a diaper, unable to sit up. She slept on an air mattress in her living room for months. I am lucky that our apartment has no stairs, but here I am, stationed on the couch, moving only for necessary trips to the bathroom, during half of which I cry.

How I got here, though, is different.

This fact brings me comfort, because it's how she got there that fixates this woman, that pins her in place. Like me, she wanted a medication-free birth. Unlike me, she arrived at the hospital before she was close to fully dilated and endured a series of interventions followed by a stalled labor, which in many cases today would result in a C-section but in her case resulted in an episiotomy. When she got home, her stitches burst and she had to be re-cut and restitched, an experience that led to long-term nerve damage and chronic pain. I can hear the woman trace the long line of decisions that she made and that others made for her, questioning: if she hadn't accepted the IV drip, would she have needed the Pitocin? Should the midwife have cut her? She wants to know: where did she go wrong?

I am sad for her, but I am relieved for myself. I don't have to live with most of these questions. This woman and I wound up in the same place, broken bodies confined to living rooms, but I had no interventions. No one cut me. This is simply what my body did, split long and jagged. There is comfort in that.

It is not worth asking what would have happened had we gone to the hospital earlier because no sign ever told us to do so, and it likely would have led to interventions that I'd be second-guessing now anyway. Had I had Pitocin and torn, I would have blamed the Pitocin. Had I had an epidural and torn, I would have blamed the epidural. I would have blamed myself.

My mother tells me, "You should have had a C-section." She had a C-section with me and a vaginal birth after cesarean (VBAC) with my sister. She says the C-section was much easier to recover from.

"There wasn't time," I say, thankful that the choice was not mine to make, thankful I will not be second-guessing myself for the rest of my life.

BIRTH STORIES, PART II

Mine is not the only complicated birth story I know. Far from it. Among just my close friends, one had a placental abruption at 30 weeks and had to be medevaced to a hospital in another state, where her baby spent the first four weeks of his life in the NICU. Another hemorrhaged following her emergency C-section and required a blood transfusion and 10 days in the ICU. Another developed gestational hypertension, which gave her migraines with aura; she had to be induced in order to avoid preeclampsia, then wound up with ongoing blood pressure issues.

The summer before I got pregnant, it was all over the news: the U.S. has the highest rate of maternal mortality in the industrialized world.

But above and beyond the issue of maternal mortality, now I learn there is another problem: "severe maternal morbidity." For every U.S. woman who dies as a consequence of pregnancy or childbirth, dozens more suffer dangerous or life-threatening complications. The CDC estimates 50,000 to 60,000 women per year. That's 135 women a day on the low end.

These are women who undergo blood transfusions, emergency hysterectomies, ventilation, and temporary tracheostomies. These are women who, during delivery, experience shock, sepsis, heart failure, and aneurysms. These numbers don't even include women like me, who, according to the hospital, have a birth without incident but are discharged with an untold number of stitches (or one long suture). My medical records from that day list five events:

- Encounter for full-term uncomplicated delivery
- Single live birth
- Third-degree perineal laceration during delivery
- Repair complex wound
- Obstetric care routine

My friends and I count ourselves lucky. Our babies made it. We made it. But two years later, listening to a few of us recount our birth stories, my friend's partner will say, "This sounds like a support group," and perhaps that is what we all need.

BEING IN THE WORLD

"When did you know you wanted to have a baby?" a friend asks.

"Truthfully," I say, a rhetorical tic I loathe but that buys me time while I try to figure out how to explain it. "Truthfully, it was the bookstore incident."

My friend knows what I am talking about.

In the spring of 2018, my mother and I took my nine-year-old niece to a bookstore and told her to pick out any book she wanted. I didn't know my niece well; my mother had recently remarried and this was the child of one of my new step-siblings. But she reminded me of myself at nine, a reader and a daydreamer, and so, on a visit home, I suggested the bookstore outing. It was a Sunday morning. My niece's mother waved us off from the front porch.

At the bookstore, we browsed the shelves and talked about our favorites: *The Devil's Arithmetic, The Westing Game*. My niece showed us a series of biographies for kids and began to list the ones she'd read. *Who Was Frida Kahlo? Who Was Jesse Owens?*

Then, as if this scene were spliced with one from another movie, there was the sound of men shouting, there were men running, there was the unreal pop of gunshots. I ducked behind an endcap while my mother threw her whole body over my niece, an instinct I instantly recognized I did not possess. The men were twenty feet away from us as they ran through the store and out into the parking lot.

I called 911. I whispered our location but immediately realized the sound of the operator's voice demanding that I speak louder might attract an active shooter, so I hung up. Barely a month had passed since Parkland, and all I could picture was the gunman walking back into the store and taking down anyone he could find.

The shooting stopped. An eerie calm set in and then was broken by a toddler's wail. A woman in a long skirt walked by me with such purpose that I thought she must be an accomplice of the shooter, until I realized that she was not down on the ground with the rest of us because it was her child, crying for her.

The bookstore was in a mall, and the whole mall went on lockdown. The bookstore manager herded us into a stockroom, all 101 of us, and we waited together for news for hours. One of the women near us worked at the Claire's upstairs and kept asking to be let out so that she could get her pump, because her breasts were painfully full. The bookstore employees, mostly teenagers, passed out cups of water. I tried to be cheerful for my niece, but all I could think about was how this day would change her.

We found out later that the shooter had not re-entered the mall; he was not looking to kill indiscriminately but rather had been aiming for a particular target, someone he knew. None of the bullets he fired hit anyone. The cop who took our names as they let us out of the stock room joked that it was lucky the guy had no aim.

Still, I heard gunshots everywhere I went, saw weapons where there were none. Every time I passed a man on the street, I flinched. I began avoiding crowds and the subway. I had a panic attack when a stranger approached me in the park to ask for directions. My mind knew that no one was killed that day; my body's response was to the sound of the gun.

"So the fact of your death became real to you," my friend says, "and it made you want to bring new life into the world?"

No. That is not it at all. "I was having such a hard time leaving the apartment, being in the world." Daniel and I used to joke that I never needed to try LSD because my natural disposition was that of a person regularly microdosing, in awe of everything. Years after the fact, he located that bookstore as the place I lost my joy. "I had all this anxiety that something bad would happen, something random and out of my control. I needed to make something happen to myself."

This is part of it, the part that is about fear and power. And then there is another part, a part about love. My mother, shielding her granddaughter with her whole body.

A STORY

"You felt so empowered while you were pregnant," my therapist reminds me.

It's true. Pregnancy was a miraculous antidote to the anxiety I'd been living with since that day in the bookstore, the reason I'd sought out therapy in the first place. Being pregnant made me feel invincible, like I had a bubble of protection around me as I walked down the street. I felt that nothing bad could happen to a pregnant woman, which is ridiculous. Bad things happen to pregnant women all the time.

But I felt safe, particularly after the 27-week mark, which is around the time a baby can generally subsist outside the womb. Should something happen, my baby stood a chance.

Before that point, there was risk. In my early twenties, I'd had two procedures to remove precancerous cervical cells, leaving me with a significantly shortened cervix. One option, my doctor explained early in the pregnancy, was to insert a prophylactic stitch that would keep my cervix from spontaneously opening too early. There was, however, the chance that the stitch itself could cause the fetus to abort.

The other option was to heavily monitor the situation and only take action if necessary. This is the road we chose, and so I had ultrasounds every two weeks, whereas most pregnant women have between zero and two total.

While each ultrasound appointment came with a certain amount of anxiety, my fears were calmed when I saw the little face, the little hands, the movement. As the appointments stacked upon one another and nothing bad happened, they began to have a soothing effect.

During the last of these precautionary ultrasounds, which ended when the fetus would have been viable outside the womb, the technician told me that—contrary to what was expected, that my short cervix would grow shorter and thinner over the course of the pregnancy—my cervix had actually doubled in length. When I asked why at that and subsequent appointments, all I got were shrugs. One nurse practitioner told me, "We know almost nothing about the cervix." Mine fulfilled its protective role, despite the traumas it had endured.

I felt strong and secure. I had a tiny companion with me at all times. No longer was I talking or singing to myself; someone was always listening. When I was a teenager, I believed I had a personal relationship with Jesus, and being pregnant was the closest I've ever come to recapturing that feeling.

"It makes what happened next all the more surprising,"

my therapist says.

But does it? A pregnant person suddenly, miraculously, feels safe and happy and protected. Surely something bad is about to happen. Or at least that's how I would read the story now.

NEED, PART I

There is one thing I wish I'd done differently.

When, ten hours into labor, I called our doula for the second time and she told me to call again when I thought I needed her, I should have said, "I am calling you now."

I second-guessed my understanding of the contractions, my decision to reach out for help at that moment. If she didn't think I should need her, then maybe I didn't really need her. Maybe I was just being needy, the act of needing too much or needing what one doesn't deserve. I was embarrassed by my neediness. I was ashamed.

I trusted her implicit assessment because she had done birth before. She was the expert. But she was not in my body. I should have said, "I need you."

It was difficult to allow for my body to be a needy, wanting thing. For those of us taught not to take up too much space, to state a need at all can be radical. Now, all I am is need, a body tended to with a hot washcloth.

Three weeks after the baby is born, though I have still barely moved from the couch, I develop a new tear. This time, I insist: something is wrong.

We go to the doctor. The new tear is minor; the doctor refers to it as an abrasion. She is reluctant to add more stitches, so she cleans the wound and I am given another round of supplies: lidocaine in aerosol cans, hydrogen peroxide to apply twice a day, epsom salt for the baths I don't have the energy to take. I return to my station on the couch and allow the mothers to take care of me.

BIRTH FATHER

In the empty space when the baby sleeps, my mother starts talking about her birth father.

When my grandmother was 25 years old and had three kids, she left her husband. Not only was he abusive, but he was an alcoholic, like her father had been. Plus, she was entangled with someone new, a semi-pro baseball player who hung around the restaurant where she worked. He had a tattoo on his bicep of a skunk holding a flower and below the skunk, drawn freehand, the word STINKY. His name was Robert, but everybody called him Duke.

I don't remember how old I was when I discovered that I was not genetically related to my Grandpa Duke. Old enough to remember my mother saying, "It doesn't matter. He raised me, he was there for us. He's my dad." Grandpa Duke formally adopted my grandmother's kids—my mother and two of her brothers—and then they had two more. Or maybe they had two more, and then he adopted the other three. I have this image of my grandmother alone for a time, single and working and trying to take care of her kids, but my mother tells me now it was messier than that.

My grandmother was pregnant, and Duke had a choice to stay or leave. He chose to stay. "She kicked her husband out and Duke moved in." That baby was born, and then they had another, two more boys.

"For a while," my mother says, "he came and picked us up on Sundays." He meaning her birth father, us meaning the three oldest kids. "We would get dressed up and wait for him in the living room. And then one day, he just stopped showing up. We sat on the couch all day and he never came."

"Why?"

"I don't know. I suspect it was because my mom told him that Duke was planning to adopt us. It was around that time. I was glad because I hated getting dressed up, but my older brother was so upset. He kept waiting for him. Every Sunday, he would put on his nice clothes and sit in the front room, waiting. He did that for a long time."

The baby monitor crackles and we both hold our breath and stare at it, my mother poised to rise and retrieve the baby from the bedroom, but no cry follows. She relaxes back into the chair.

"Were you sad?"

"No, things got better after Duke moved in. There was no more physical fighting, no more cops being called." She pauses and reconsiders. "Well, their fights came later."

I have heard about these fights, passionate battles that often resulted in my grandmother disappearing, sometimes for days at a time. I have heard how Grandpa Duke would trail her in his car as she stomped down the highway, how he would beg her to get back in. "Babe," I can hear him say. "Mare," short for Mary, short for Magdeline.

"My older brother found our birth father. Went and visited him a few years ago. He was living in a trailer not too far away. When he died, he left my brother twenty thousand dollars. Nothing for his other kids. Nothing for my mom, who was owed years of child support. Grandpa Duke kept a ledger for years, kept track of every penny my mom was owed."

This is the most I have ever heard my mother talk about her birth father. It is as if the baby has unlocked something in her. Birth is a portal that can take us to other births. Newborns are portals to the people who came before them, back when those young lives were still made up of possibilities.

AN ABRIDGED SEARCH HISTORY, PART II

4 weeks postpartum still heavy bleeding
postpartum bladder pressure
postpartum pelvic pressure
postpartum bruising
postpartum itching
postpartum constipation when to see doctor
how to poop with an anal tear
sharp anal pain
what to do with a baby all day
when do babies get teeth
baby grunting in sleep
baby seems uncomfortable on back
how to put baby back to sleep
pelvic floor therapy brooklyn ny

THE LAYING OF HANDS

Like the birth story, this story can also be told for comic effect.

When the baby is four weeks old and my sister is staying with us, caring for me and the baby while Daniel is at work, my body succumbs to the copious amounts of ibuprofen I have been consuming—600 milligrams every four hours, often on an empty stomach because I am afraid to eat—and becomes constipated. I am still taking daily laxatives and stool softeners, things that are supposed to make bowel movements easier to allow the tear to heal, but for a few days nothing happens. With each day that passes, my fear grows: the more time goes by, the more painful it will be.

By Saturday morning, I am in agony. I have to go, but I can't go. I describe the feeling to my sister, who listens and rubs my back as if I am one of her own children. My sister tries to live her life like Jesus, and in moments of crisis, it really shows.

I resolve that I will try again. I make my way slowly from the living room to the bathroom, a walk that still takes so much energy, and sit on the toilet, waiting. I have been warned not to strain, been told to simply breathe deeply from my belly and let it happen.

When finally there is movement, at first I am relieved. Then the pain hits and I feel my body shaken by a large hand, an uncontrollable scream jolted from me, the low moan underneath it taking me right back to the backseat of the car, trying to hold the baby in. It feels like I am shitting shards of glass.

My sister comes running at the sound of my screams. "It's worse than labor," I tell her.

I make my way to bed and google what to do. Google tells me to use a laxative suppository, and so Daniel goes to the pharmacy to get one. I lie in bed moaning while my sister takes care of the baby, which reminds me there is a baby. My head is foggy. I am certain that my body is being poisoned from the inside by the waste in my gut. I am willing to try anything.

The laxative suppository is medicine encased in a lump of fat shaped like a bullet. The directions say to slide it into the rectum and hold it in for twenty minutes. I lie on my side and push it inside me, where it burns. Again, I feel the need to go, and again it results in nothing but tortuous pain. I stumble back to bed to cry and writhe. My sister asks if she can pray for me and though it's been fifteen years since I last prayed myself, I nod. She asks for healing, she asks for rest.

I call my OBGYN's weekend line, the one for medical

emergencies, and reach the owner of the practice in his car, his voice over Bluetooth far away. He tells me to try a second suppository, and if that doesn't work, to go to the emergency room. He tells me that when it is not the weekend, I will need a gastroenterologist, someone who specializes in this problem. The injury may have been caused by birth, but I am now outside the realm of birth. I feel he is washing his hands of me.

The second suppository does not work, and so we head to the ER: Daniel, the baby, my sister, and me.

Bringing a four-week old baby to a New York City ER is a bad idea, but we don't know what else to do. The hospital is twenty minutes away, more with traffic, and I am breastfeeding every two to three hours. Daniel waits with the baby in the waiting room while my sister accompanies me through the large door, where I am told I will receive an enema. Getting an enema while recovering from a third-degree tear sounds like a terrible idea, but, again, we don't know what else to do.

In the ER, hospital beds are lined up in close quarters, separated by hanging curtains. There is an old woman on the other side of our curtain who can't breathe and whose stomach hurts. She keeps saying, "I don't want to go like this." The nurse stationed at the end of our two beds ignores her. Another nurse walking by hears her and offers her water. She is terrified, and I am terrified for her.

The enema is ordered right away, but the wait for it is hours. At some point, I make my way slowly to the waiting room to feed the baby. Standing is painful but sitting is unthinkable, so I feed him standing up for as long as I can bear it, long enough to satisfy his cries, then return to the hospital bed to wait some more. Three nurses at a central nurses' station flirt, and I feel happy for them that they have something to look forward to at work but also wonder if their patients are, like me, waiting in pain for help. My sister tries to find the doctor who examined me, but he is gone. She flags down a different doctor, one who looks kind and turns out to be. He looks into it. Somewhere along the way, there was a miscommunication. The enema was ordered but no one has been told to administer it.

The nurse stationed at the end of the bed is selected for the honor. She is rough, and I sob. She numbs me with lidocaine and tells me to hold the enema solution in for as long as possible, otherwise she may have to do it again. The solution begins to work and I feel as if I will explode. Surely there will be no me after this. Now I am made of tears and breast milk and shit.

That is when my sister lays hands. Gently, she touches me and begins to speak softly in tongues. I know the sound immediately, the sibilance and soft clicking. Part of me is embarrassed: my sister, interceding on my behalf to ask God to help me poop, right there in front of the nurses and doctors and other patients. But it is so surreal and I am so desperate for relief from my pain that another part of me welcomes it and I am able to close my eyes and experience my sister's inscrutable prayers for what they are: intense love.

When I can't take it any longer, my sister guides me to a single-person bathroom where I am finally able to empty my insides. My whole body shakes as I say, "I'm sorry, I'm sorry, I'm sorry," because the stink of it is unbearable. My sister rubs my back and tells me it's okay, and she means it.

My adult diaper is filled with lochia and blood, so my sister goes to request a fresh pad. I suddenly realize how long it's been since I've showered, how sweaty I am. A mosquito buzzes around the bathroom and I don't have the energy to do anything but observe it and hope it does not land on me. My sister lets herself back into the bathroom and hands me the pad. She spots the mosquito and kills it with one hand.

WORSE THAN LABOR

"It wasn't really worse than labor," Daniel says later, reminding me how I cried as I vomited between contractions.

But it was worse, in part because it was more terrifying. Labor is supposed to hurt. When labor is painful, the body does not automatically sound its death alarm.

"It was," I say, but it is difficult to explain how the layer of fear makes the pain count double, how the weeks of constant pain pile atop one another, making any new pain exponentially worse. When I delivered my baby, I was ripped open once. Now, I am being ripped open continually.

THE FIRST FORTY DAYS

While I was waiting for the baby to arrive, I read a handful of books about pregnancy and birth. These books are full of checklists and plans, and reading them helped me to feel more in control. I read Ina May Gaskin's *Spiritual Midwifery* and envisioned my own ecstatic birth. I read a how-to-birth book that recommended we bring twinkle lights, music, and essential oils to the hospital, all things that we packed that never made it out of the hospital bag. Some of these books suggested ludicrous rituals like lining up one's friends with children on one side of a room and one's childless friends on the other and then, heavy with symbolism and the woven flower crown on one's head, crossing from one side to the other, an exercise which would have done nothing but lose me friends.

Many of these books talk about the first forty days postpartum as a sacred time of healing, pointing to various traditions across cultures of sitting or lying in, often surrounded by the women in one's family. They describe the intense healing process the body must go through after birth: the wound, left by the placenta, that is the size of a dinner plate; the shedding of mucus and blood as the uterus shrinks back to its original size, watermelon to clenched fist. They encourage foods dense in nutrients like liver, fish stock, and oxtails, long-simmering dishes made by loving aunts who know how to cook. I consumed book after book, as if reading them would magically bring those aunts into my life or extend my parental leave. I wish now I'd spent that time reading poetry; I would have been better prepared.

None of the books I read described pain so intense that I would not be able to move. None discussed how to have a bowel movement without bursting my stitches. None told me what to do if forty days came and went and I still was not healed.

RASPBERRIES

People bring food: pizza, bagels, ice cream. I don't touch any of it.

I am terrified of eating because I know what will happen when the food becomes waste. Every bite I put in my mouth is calculated based on what will give me the most nutrients for breastfeeding while causing the least pain on the way out. For months I subsist mainly on three meals: smoothies, the homemade lactation "cookies" I made and froze before the birth, and oatmeal with raspberries.

I order the raspberries via an app on my phone and they show up every few days, pints and pints of them. I have never spent so much money on fruit, but the raspberries feel safe in a way that no other food does. I eat so many raspberries that the baby's poop starts to smell like raspberries. For years, I will associate the smell of raspberries with the liquid smear in the baby's diaper, which my sister changes as I watch from the couch.

HOLD ON

I apply an oil called Nourish & Replenish to my face once a day. It helps me retain some sense of my old life, of my body alive.

I shuffle from the living room to the bathroom, bent severely at the waist, wincing the whole way. I pee, holding the edges of the toilet to steady myself through the pain. I wash my hands slowly, noticing the ritual of it but finding my mind too clouded to think anything beyond that. Then I squeeze five drops of the oil from a dropper into my palm and mix it with a mineral mist. I massage it into my cheeks, my chin, the bridge of my nose. It smells of holy basil and reminds me of my life.

I have nowhere to go. No one is looking at my skin. This is an oil I have requested for Christmas every year for the last decade, an oil I hoard throughout the year because it is by far the priciest personal care item I own. Now, I spend it all. I tip my head back slowly and rub the oil into my neck. I face myself in the mirror and turn my head side to side, see my skin glisten. This is one way I hold on.

MOM AND BABY

A casual friend gives birth.

Mom and baby are healthy and happy, the group text reads.

These are words I now find suspect, as if the whole thing is one big cover-up.

"But how are you *doing*?" I ask new moms meaningfully. "How are *you* doing?"

HOLDING, PART II

Eventually, I do begin to second-guess.

Just after the birth, the woman who taught our birth class emailed to ask how we are. She was mostly interested in how breastfeeding was going, whether we needed a lactation consultation. I told her all the good news—feeding is going great! We're getting more sleep than we thought we would! Keeping a cheery tone, I briefly mentioned the injury. Her response seemed, at first, incongruous to me.

Home birth next time ;)

I replied with three laughing crying faces and quickly moved on.

Now, I wonder if a home birth might have resulted in a better outcome.

I look up risk factors for my injury.

- ☑ First birth
- 🛇 High birth weight
- 🛇 Shoulder dystocia
- 🛇 Occipito-posterior position

? Prolonged second stage of labor
⊘ Instrumental delivery

I wonder if the long drive to the hospital, during which I was likely fully dilated, the exasperated negotiations with the hospital attendant who tried to get me to sit me in a wheelchair when I had a baby's head between my legs, the brief journey from the hospital's sliding doors to the delivery room where I was finally given permission to let go of my hold on the baby—I wonder if this holding was what tore me. If we had only gone to the hospital earlier. If we had only had the baby at home. If we had only let the baby come when the baby was ready to come.

NEED, PART II

When my sister has to go home to tend to her own children but I am still not able to lift the baby or care for him on my own, my mother offers to fly out again to stay with us for a second time. This is more help than we had asked for or planned on before the birth, and I find it difficult to say yes. There must be someone else I could call upon. Do I need my mother? I'm not sure. Do I want her? Yes.

She arrives and I am relieved. This time I am well enough to talk, to prop myself up to nearly sitting. The baby sleeps on us, in our arms or draped over our outstretched legs. My mother speaks softly, lovingly to him and I try to imagine her doing the same to me when I was a baby, but it's not an image I can conjure. When my mother remembers me as a baby, she remembers how sick I was, how loud and long I cried, how stubbornly I refused to be soothed. How I was colicky and prone to infections.

My mother had a difficult birth, a long and painful labor that ended in emergency C-section. I was in the NICU for 10 days, my mother separated from her baby while her body recovered from the shock and her milk dried up. She went back to work after four weeks, not unusual then or now.

I try to imagine being back at work. I cannot yet walk or stand straight without pain. I cannot carry my baby from one room to the other, can only hold him if someone places him in my arms. Perhaps my mind could do the work, but at what cost to my body? My stitches are not fully dissolved. I am yet an open wound.

While we are sitting and talking and looking at the baby, my mother receives a notification from my grandmother's medical alert system. She is third in line, which means my Grandpa Duke and the uncle who lives closest to my grandparents have already been notified and have not responded.

I can feel my mother's worry in my own body, a tense wire running through me. She calls my grandparents' landline, my grandpa's cell phone, multiple times with no response. Finally, she reaches my uncle, who received the life alert while undergoing dental work and left the dentist's chair to rush to my grandparents' house.

My grandmother has fallen. She has hit her face on the coffee table. She is bruised and bloodied. Her nose may be broken.

They are still on the phone when my grandpa comes home and a screaming match ensues. My grandmother is not supposed to be left alone, and where was he? The post office. What business does he have at the post office? What must he mail? My mother holds the phone away from her face, listens as her dad and her brother argue while her mother bleeds.

My grandmother is taken to the hospital. My mother, doing all she can from afar, calls ahead to let the ER know they are coming.

My mother is anguished: she has flown across the country to care for her daughter, but now her own mother back home needs her. One day, I will be her. One day, it will be her own need that I feel beyond the mountains that lie between us.

A LITERAL NAZI

My mother refers to her great-grandfather as a Nazi, a term she has used to describe him before.

"Was he really a Nazi?" I ask. I am sitting in a chair, nursing the baby. Not sitting, exactly; my legs are folded under me and I am leaning on the armrest because it will be a long time before my butt can actually touch a chair, but still. We are waiting for an update on my grandmother's condition, and it is that or perhaps the fact that I made a baby with a Jewish man that brings my great-great-grandfather to my mother's mind.

"Of course he was." My mother is sitting on the couch that I exclusively have occupied since the baby was born, the couch that is no longer relegated to being a sickbed.

"I always thought when you called him a Nazi, you meant that he was a bad man."

"He was a bad man." My mother's face contorts at the ugly thought of him. "He was a bad, bad man. A terrible man."

I know that he was a bad man. The previous summer, while she was visiting New York and we were wearing the matching orange Moms Demand Action T-shirts I had bought us, my mother confided in me that this man had sexually abused several girls in the family, including her and almost certainly including my grandmother.

I am starting to feel pain, but I am determined to remain upright until the baby is done nursing. "But he came over before the party was founded. He wasn't a literal Nazi."

"You know he gave away his daughter?"

I know this part of the story. My great-great-grandfather, the Nazi, was at fault in a car accident that caused an acquaintance, a man named Frank, to lose his leg. In order to make it up to Frank, my great-great-grandfather, the Nazi, offered one of his daughters to be Frank's wife. Frank requested Susie, but Susie ran off and married someone else, so he wound up with Helen, the youngest. She was fourteen.

Frank was Helen's father's age; like her father, he had been born in the old country around the turn of the century. He was already an alcoholic at the time of the car accident, and his injury only exacerbated his drinking problem. The marriage was not a happy one.

And neither was it a long one. When Frank died of his alcoholism, Helen abandoned their three young children, my grandmother and her two brothers. The children were split up and raised by different family members. My grandmother wound up with the Nazi and his wife.

It was an unhappy life that my grandmother escaped by dropping out of high school and marrying young herself, but at the end of the Nazi's life, when he was old and sick, she surprised everybody by taking him in.

"I was thirteen when his wife died and he moved in with us," my mother continues. "He used to sit in his room and scream at the television newscasters. 'Dirty fucking Jews!'" She imitates his Austrian accent.

The baby lets go of my right breast and I sit him up to burp him. I am just now learning to do this simple task of mothering; other people have been burping the baby for me. I am unsure and feel as if I might drop or inadvertently choke him.

"We would all say, 'Why is he here?'"

The baby's head slumps forward. I am doing it wrong.

"She moved him into our house, after he raped his own step-daughter, after what he did to her. She brought him into our house."

"Why?"

My mother thinks about this. "Maybe she felt she owed it to her grandmother, who took her in when she had no one else."

FAMILY SECRETS

My grandmother does not know what happened to my mother at the hands of the Nazi. When she asked my mother if he'd ever touched her, my mother lied and said no.

"Why did you lie?" I asked my mother when she told me.

"There was a psychiatrist there," my mother said. At some point during one of my grandmother's stints in rehab, a group counseling session had been recommended and reluctantly withstood. "Grandpa Duke was there. I didn't want to get into it. And I didn't think it would help anybody."

This is the kind of secret that poisons a family slowly, over decades, the kind that I felt long before I was told. It shaped the way my grandmother raised my mother, the way my mother raised me and my sister. If I let it, it will touch my baby, too.

But my grandmother must know. Otherwise, she wouldn't have asked.

SAFE

My mother and I decide to take the baby out for a walk. We are only in the elevator of my building when I begin to think I will not make it. Standing, even tilted forward at the hips, I feel my organs weighing down on me, threatening to fall out of me. There is a lemon poking out of my vagina, scraping against my underwear, and every step pushes it down, down, down. I pause, bend fully forward to put my hands on my knees and release some of the pressure. I breathe. I want to make it.

My mother is pushing the baby in the stroller. I think that we are glacial, and then I wonder what my son will learn of glaciers, how they were ruined by the people who came before him. I reach out to put a hand on the push bar when I think I might fall.

We make it to the crosswalk at the end of our block and, although we have the walk sign, I stop to gather my strength.

Before I am ready to proceed, an SUV comes speeding down the wrong side of the road, passing all the cars at the stoplight, blowing through the red and peeling out in a left turn. Though we are on the sidewalk still, the vehicle comes dangerously close to the stroller. Had we been just one step into the crosswalk, we would have been hit.

Another SUV comes close behind it and pulls the same move, followed shortly thereafter by a sedan. I miss the driver of the first car, but I see the driver of the second and the look on his face terrifies me: angry, determined. He is not looking at us.

The driver of the car sitting obediently in the left turn lane, waiting for the light to change, rolls down his window and leans out. "Something's going down," he shouts at us. "You should go inside."

We should go inside. Because we are two women, out on our own. Because we have a tiny baby in a stroller. Because I am clearly frail, sickly.

We turn and scuttle back into our building, the pain of moving quickly almost more than I can bear but the fear of violence pushing me to get my baby inside, away from it.

When we are inside, my mother says, "He had a gun."

"Who had a gun?"

"The second driver."

"I didn't see a gun."

"I saw it. He was holding it with one hand and steering

with the other."

This is not what I think I saw, but it happened so quickly.

I often see guns where there are probably not guns. I understand why my mother would, too.

My mother is worried about the neighborhood.

"It's safe," I say, but what guarantees can I make? No place feels safe to me anymore. "I've never seen anything like that here before," I say, which is true. "This is a neighborhood where people come to raise their kids," I say. When there are enough mothers, there will be no more guns, I reason to myself. I want to believe.

CRYING

At the six-week postpartum visit, I am asked to fill out a questionnaire that will tell the doctor whether I have postpartum depression. The questionnaire asks how often I have cried for no reason.

I know what it feels like to cry for "no reason," to shed tears that I have trouble connecting to a particular thought or feeling. I know what it feels like to cry over an idea that is clear to me but is also irrational, to experience worry ungrounded in reality. To cycle through feelings from past experiences as if they are happening again, happening always. Sometimes I just need to cry. Pressure builds up, some word or tone of voice turns a valve, tears come out. There is an element of release.

Since the birth, I have cried every day. I have cried because I was sad. I have cried because I was disappointed. I have cried because I was in physical pain.

For once in my life, my tears are easy to explain. I check the box that says NEVER.

MY BABY

Someone tells me that I will feel like shit for a long time, and then one day I will wake up and feel better. Not one hundred percent better, maybe not even eighty percent better, but better. And it's true: one day, around six weeks after the birth, I find I can walk from the couch to the bathroom standing not fully upright, but nearly. Soon, I am able to hold the baby standing up if someone places him in my arms, and not long after that, I am strong enough to carry him from the living room to the bedroom. The baby begins to feel like my baby.

I am horrified by the thought of what would have happened if I had been alone, with no one to care for the baby or for me.

"You would have done what you needed to do to take care of the baby," my mother says.

But I wouldn't have. I couldn't have. I realize that even the people who took care of me, who brought me water and broth and oatmeal, who watched me struggle to bend my knees or lift myself up onto my elbows, do not understand how far inside myself I had to retreat during those early weeks in order to simply keep my body going. If it had been just the two of us, I don't think I could have done it for the baby, too.

LEAVE, PART II

The caregivers return to their own homes, and I am left with the baby while Daniel works. Four weeks remain of my leave from work, and I am still barely able to go outside the apartment. I change my first diaper. I let the baby nap on my body, partly because he is most easily soothed this way and partly because the effort of carrying him to the bedroom and lowering him into the bassinet is too taxing. I read out loud to him *The Talented Mr. Ripley* and *Goodbye, Columbus.*

I begin to take a daily walk to the end of the block and back, the baby in the stroller and my steps slow and halting. After a few more weeks, I grow braver and try carrying him on my body in a cotton wrap, but the extra pressure on my pelvic floor causes me to wet myself.

The leave I had imagined—bonding with my baby, meeting up with friends in coffee shops, trying "mommy and me" yoga once and then deciding it's not for me—is not a possibility, and I grieve for it. My days are still consumed by horrifying bathroom trips, nightly sitz baths that are supposed to be healing but that leave me itchy and uncomfortable, and a near-paralyzing fear of moving too quickly or in the wrong direction. I am still in pain, and the pain scares me because I'm not sure if it's normal.

Surrounding my sense of loss is a secondary feeling of guilt; I judge myself for being sad. The baby is healthy, the baby is growing, the baby smiles his first smile. I should be grateful, and I try. I keep a cheery log of milestones: Baby loves kisses on the cheek! Baby doesn't like gas! But I worry that the baby can sense that this is not how things were supposed to go.

A VISITATION

My friend Heather offers to bike to my apartment to cut my hair. Normally, I go to her. I am miles out of her way, but I have not had a haircut in months, so though it feels like a lot to ask, I say yes.

"I know how tough it is to leave with a new baby," she says.

Heather does not have kids, but her sister does, and she has the kind of relationship with her sister that involves a lot of empathy: she is fiercely on her sister's side. And so she understands the challenges of the postpartum period without having gone through it herself, a rarity. I am not the kind of person who could have put myself in these shoes hypothetically, but Heather is. Despite this, I have yet to tell her about the injury, which I will now try to manage long enough to sit in a chair for the length of a haircut.

She arrives and it feels like what it is: an enormous generosity. I put the baby in his bouncer and rock him with my foot while she arranges a mirror so that I can see myself. I will him to fall asleep, but he's wide awake. She runs her fingers through my hair and asks what I'm thinking.

I am thinking that I don't look like myself. I am as thin

as I was at the height of my eating-disordered early twenties, and my hair is longer than it's ever been: shoulder-length and plain, no fringe or fun undercut. I let it all grow out during the pregnancy so that I could put it in a ponytail after the baby was born. People told me there would be no time to shower.

I don't recognize myself, but Heather seems to, and this is another generosity.

I met Heather years ago at the salon where she used to work. I called for an appointment with whoever and got her, a person who will ask the near-stranger in her chair questions about life and death, a person with a full sleeve of tattoos featuring a red octopus with a monocle reading a book, a person who will remember your hopes and dreams and ask about them the next time, who will gently hold you accountable to going after them. By the time Heather left the salon, we were friends. She began cutting my hair out of her apartment, which is where she also taught me about tarot and gave me my first deck, a well-loved Waite-Smith.

As Heather snips my hair and the dead ends fall to the ground, she asks me how I am and I tell her the story—the full story—of the birth and its aftermath.

The baby begins to fuss so I rock the bouncer harder. I tell Heather how bad it's been, how bad it still is. She doesn't give me advice or try to fix anything. She simply listens as she shapes me into something more recognizable, pausing occasionally to look at my eyes in the mirror and let me know she hears. When she is done with the cut, I feel as if a tiny part of my trouble lies on the floor with the clippings. She sweeps it away with a broom.

I want Heather to stay all day, I want to soak up her calm energy, but the baby starts to wail. She hugs me goodbye, and I am alone again with the baby.

TABOO

When I can finally venture out of the apartment, I am astounded by the number of people—friends, acquaintances, strangers—who comment on my weight. They think this is okay, because I lost all my pregnancy weight immediately, plus some.

They tell me how skinny I am, look at the tiny baby in Daniel's arms and then look my body up and down. They scrutinize my torso and say things like, "Are you sure there was a baby in there?" One person tells me I look better than before I got pregnant.

The worst is when other mothers compare my body to their own, pat their bellies and say things like, "I had my kid three years ago and look at me." As if it were a contest, as if I should be ecstatic that I won.

These people see me as lucky, but the cause of my weight loss is invisible and ongoing, and talking about it is taboo.

Sometimes I attempt to make a joke. "You try blowing open your asshole and see if you want to eat." Other times I strike a more serious note. "I am having a difficult recovery process." Both approaches make people uncomfortable. They are simply trying, misguided, to pay me a compliment. Finally, I land on saying nothing at all.

PHOTOS

I return to the photographs of the birth. We don't have many; we thought there would be time that there was not.

They begin at 8:32 in the morning, when I am fairly certain I'm in early labor and decide to go for a walk. I pose before the mirror in the lobby of our building. I am wearing athletic shorts with a maternity workout tank top and nursing sports bra. In one hand is a water bottle that I bought specifically for the birth, because the woman who taught our birth class insisted we would need a water bottle with a straw. In the other is a medical bill in its return envelope, stamped and ready to drop in a post box.

The next two photos are from 6:59pm. The bedroom lights are off, but the hall light is on and twilight comes from the windows. I am sitting on a blue yoga ball, also purchased for the birth. My workout clothes have come off. I sit in my underwear and sports bra, holding my belly with a hand on either side of my protruding navel. In the first of these photos, I am taking in a breath, eyes closed, my lips in the slightest smile. In the second, I am letting out the breath, slow and controlled like I have been taught. My eyes are open and locked on someone off camera. It is me, in the mirror.

There is a short series of photos taken by the doula in the moments just after the baby's birth at 9:58pm. My legs are open wide and the baby, covered in vernix, is being handed up to me by gloved hands. Daniel stands next to the bed, looking happy and relieved. The look on my face is a cross between joy and terror.

The photos after this are of the baby on my chest. The nursing flaps of the sports bra have come down and my exposed breast takes up most of each photo until the photographer, Daniel, decides to change the angle. Then there is the baby, using my breast as a pillow, looking up at nothing. I am smiling.

What, now, am I searching for? Some sign on someone's face that something is wrong? Some new piece of information or lost memory? Evidence—but of what?

In one photo, there is a reflection in the window of the giant circular surgical light by which the doctor is assessing the damage, preparing to begin her stitching. I don't remember the light, but I do remember that everything felt too bright.

GENERATIONS

When the baby is seven weeks old, my mother calls to tell me that my grandmother's brother has died.

"She is the last one," my mother says, meaning the last of her generation.

But my grandmother is not the last one. She has a set of much younger half-siblings. My great-grandmother, Helen, eventually settled down, married, had a real family, with children she wanted. When my grandmother was pregnant with my mother, her own mother was pregnant, too.

The fracture in our family means I don't know this great-uncle who has died, and I didn't know the one who died before him. Of my grandmother's half-siblings, the only one whose name I know is Evie, a woman I met once, at a funeral when I was in high school. I don't even know how many there are.

"How is she?" I ask my mother.

The death has been difficult for her emotionally. Physically, she is doing a little better. Her face is healing. There was a medical inquiry into the cause of the fall, but we all knew what it would turn up: a medley of painkillers, my grandmother's own special recipe. For a brief time after the last emergency room visit, my mother held out hope that this would be a turning point, but it seems to have had the opposite effect. Now there are new prescriptions to treat the physical pain from the fall; now when I call, my grandmother, who has never had a drink in her life, sounds wasted and far away.

DRUG SEEKERS

In my twenties, I worked in customer service at a healthcare technology startup, and this job put me in the way of doctors daily. Through a headset, I spoke with doctors who were unhappy with their online reviews, who wanted those reviews to be washed away. They would call about a two-star review with no comments. Though the review was anonymous, they insisted they knew who left it. That patient was a drug seeker, they would say.

Drug-seeking patient. So many of them said it that I knew instinctively it was a term of art. A label that perfectly described my grandmother. A label that, to many of the doctors I spoke with, meant the person didn't deserve to leave a review of their appointment, couldn't provide a fair evaluation of a physician's bedside manner or the wait time at the office. A label that meant they weren't a real patient.

The problem of the drug-seeking patient was part of my interview for the job. It was presented as a puzzle: The same patient has booked multiple upcoming appointments, all on the same day and all with different doctors who practice the same specialty: pain medicine. What should we do?

The correct answer, according to the interview script, is

to assume positive intent while finding a technological solution to the problem.

Perhaps the patient is just trying to find the right doctor—someone close to her, at a time that works for her schedule—and is having trouble canceling the appointments she doesn't want.

Perhaps the patient is trying to book for herself and her family but is having trouble creating additional accounts.

Perhaps the patient wants a second opinion, and a third.

(Perhaps the patient is an opioid addict.)

This was 2012, five years before the United States Department of Health and Human Services declared the opioid epidemic a public health emergency. I had grown up witnessing my grandmother's addiction, but I had yet to connect that experience with any larger system or pattern, so I had trouble following the question, all that was implied when the interviewer landed heavily on "pain medicine." But the drug-seeking patient would become a part of my daily routine. The calls from frustrated doctors who were paying for a service that was only delivering them "drug seekers." The calls from frustrated patients who were locked out of their accounts because they had booked too many upcoming appointments. With the latter, it was up to us to determine whether the patient had a legitimate reason for hitting the appointment limit, in which case we could unlock the account, or was a likely drug seeker, in which case we were supposed to blame it on the system.

It was almost two years before one of these patients reminded me of my grandmother, but when it happened, I couldn't help but hear her voice in my headset with every locked account call, couldn't help but get defensive when doctors spoke disparagingly of people like her. Yes, she is seeking drugs, I wanted to say. But maybe she is seeking something else, too.

THE DOLL ROOM

In my grandmother's house, there is a room full of dolls. At some point in the 90s, she directed my Grandpa Duke to install shelving on every wall, from the floor to the ceiling, to display her growing collection. She ordered the dolls from infomercials and sought them out at garage sales, estate sales, and auctions. They are all porcelain and life-like, with shining glass eyes and frilly lace dresses. Most are one to two feet tall, although occasionally she splurged on a larger one or fell for a miniature. Some are baby dolls, and others are little women dressed up according to a theme: The Black Widow, The Fairy Queen, The Huntress. Each doll came with a certificate of authenticity for the collector, but my grandmother doesn't care about their provenance.

"Why does she keep buying dolls?" I asked my mother when the doll room reached its limit and the dolls began to pile up in the hallway and the dining room.

"All she wanted when she was little was a doll," my mother said. "And she never got one."

GIRL BABY

A month or two before I got pregnant, my sister told me that she had a dream, a vision from God, that I was pregnant and that the baby was a girl. When I called her to tell her I was pregnant, she said, "I know, and the baby is a girl."

It was easy for me to picture that the thing growing inside me was a girl. I grew up with a sister. I was raised in a matriarchal family. But the idea of mothering a girl made me anxious.

I began recounting in therapy the mundane failures of my mother—what I perceived to be her lack of acceptance of everything from my appearance to my life choices—and feeling, for the first time, anger at her. "You said in our very first session that your relationship with your mother was complicated," my therapist reminded me. "Good, but complicated."

The truth was, I wanted our relationship to be good, and it upset me to feel anything but love for a woman who had done her best with me.

At home over the holidays, not yet showing, I went to coffee with my sister and as soon as I brought up our mother, I began to cry. My sister passed me napkins to stem the flow of tears as I listed all the defects I felt I had inherited from the women in our family and would surely pass down to a girl: perfectionism, disordered eating, anxiety, depression.

My sister got it. Her first child was a boy and that made it easy, she said, to see her relationship to him outside of our family dynamics. It was its own new thing. But when she found out her second would be a girl, she also broke down crying, right there in the sonogram appointment. She didn't understand why. She had to process her own anger at our mother.

"How did you do it?" I was desperate to know.

My sister said that at some point, a few years back, she sat down with our mother and told her why she was angry, and our mother apologized and asked for forgiveness. My sister forgave her. As my sister described their reconciliation, I realized that she was angry about a whole different set of wrongs, things that had happened after I left home, things I had never thought twice about, some things I never even knew about. I was ready to be indignant on my sister's behalf, but she spoke about the wrongdoings with grace. She really had forgiven.

The other thing that helped, she said, was considering her own children in a generational context.

"Think about Grandma," my sister said. "Abandoned

by her mother, sexually abused by her grandfather. High school dropout. Married at seventeen, pregnant at eighteen. Physically abused by her first husband.

"Then think about Mom. Her birth father left, she was sexually abused by her great-grandfather. But she graduated from high school, she went to college, she started her own business.

"Now consider the two of us. Our childhoods were not perfect, but they were the most stable yet, and we are stronger because of it. Think about the homes we are building for our children. How much better off they'll be."

How far away from the heart of the hurt that has infected our family for a century or more.

Still, I worried that I would fuck up a girl, and I felt relief when the ultrasound technician said she saw a penis. My sister was unruffled by the news and what it meant about her vision. She suggested that perhaps there was a second baby coming.

But the girl baby was never a real baby; the girl baby was me.

GOOD DAUGHTERS

My mother tells me her oldest brother has started going to therapy. He wants her to go with him.

"Are you going to go?" I ask. (This is over the phone. We have been arguing, those same old hurts that bubble to the surface every now and again. "You're so critical of me," she says, and I say, "You're so critical of me." We are both right.)

"No," she says. "I don't want to be angry with my mom at the end of her life."

I am surprised that she can so easily identify the feeling that is waiting for her. "Why are you angry with your mom?" A question I long to ask all honest daughters.

"Because she left us at home to be abused. She invited that man into our house." The literal Nazi. "She knew what he was. And then she went to work. She left us with him."

The conversation has evolved. She is no longer proud of the fact that her mother worked, which is the narrative I remember from when I was young. Now she feels abandoned.

"I had to raise her kids. I was the one." My mother pulls

back. She does not want to be angry with her mom. "I should have gone to see my birth father before he died," she says. "She kept us from him, and then I refused to see him. No one deserves that."

This is also, according to my memory, a rewriting. "He hit her," I remind my mother, but she does not seem to hear me. "Maybe therapy would be good for you. You might be angry at first, but you can work through it. You two can have a better relationship, more honest." Now I am talking about me, now I am talking about us and all my hopes.

"No," she says. "I'm not going to turn on her at the end of her life."

For as long as I've been alive, she has been convinced that her mother is about to die. And for all those years, she has been what she thinks is a good daughter, a good daughter at the end of one's life.

DEVASTATED

“Your mother can never read this,” Daniel says.

I am surprised at his reaction. On the spectrum of caring what other people think, I am usually at the “very much” end and he is nowhere to be found.

“Why not?”

“She will be devastated.”

My first feeling is shame, but I resist. “What makes you say that?”

Daniel looks at me like I should know, but I don’t.

“Specifically, what do you think will devastate her?”

“The part about not wanting to have a girl?”

And at this I laugh, relieved. “That? No one would understand that better than my mother.”

WARMTH

"I wonder about the physicality of the speaker's mother with her," my agent says via email. "In scenes with the sister we see physical comforting, but the mother character feels distant in a way that I'm not sure how to read."

"If I were somebody reading this, I wouldn't like my character very much," my mother says.

I am hard on her because we are so alike; in her I see the stubborn taproots of my own worst faults.

With my mother's permission, I record one of our conversations. We talk for three hours. Afterward, the app I used sends me the recording, a 61-page transcript, and a list of "key" words.

worry
weird
disordered
eating
girls
felt
thought
mother

died
happy

"I wish you would remember the times I cuddled, soothed, spoke softly to you," my mother says.

This hurt hits close to home; now that I have begun caring for my own baby, my worry is that it's too late—that the emotional distance I felt at the beginning created an invisible, permanent chasm between us.

I remember sleeping on the floor next to my mother. She preferred to sleep there on cold nights so she could huddle near the floor register and trap the heat under her blanket. I remember her putting one leg over my small body in her sleep. I remember being willing to be smothered by her in order to be close, to share her warmth.

NEED PART, III

I let the baby cry for the time it takes to pee and wash my hands. I find it surprisingly easy to ignore my baby's cries, perhaps because I still think of him as part of me, and I have subjugated my own needs for so long. We can wait. We are fine. Do not worry about us.

When I pick him up, he clings to me, wails as if broken, buries his face in my chest.

What if I had let him cry for five minutes, ten? Twenty? He would still take comfort in me when I came back. This is how we are with our mothers: no matter how they let us down, abandon us, we want them when they return.

"You left out the part about how happy you were to be mothered by her," Daniel says. "When she came back the second time."

Did I? I said I wanted her. The truth is I needed her.

HOLDING, PART III

At eight weeks postpartum, I begin weekly sessions with a pelvic floor therapist. She puts her fingers inside me and gently works the scar tissue to make it softer, looser. My body has seized up and her job is to help it let go.

She is an Orthodox woman with four kids of her own, so when she tells me that I will not always pee myself when going on short walks, that it will not always feel like there is a lemon poking out of my vagina, I believe her.

Still, I am terrified by what my fingers find when I probe what the stitches have left behind. A bulge where there shouldn't be one, as if my organs have become too heavy to hold up.

It's a prolapse, the pelvic floor therapist explains: my bladder dropping down into my vaginal cavity.

"Absolutely no baby wearing," she says.

No carrying the baby beyond what is absolutely required. No lifting heavy objects. Complete this series of exercises every night before bed.

I obey, willing the routine to hold me together.

STITCHED, PART II

On YouTube, I watch videos demonstrating surgical techniques for third- and fourth-degree tear repair. Disembodied latex-gloved hands stitch pieces of thin foam together using a needle shaped like a hook, pinched between the claws of a needle holder. One layer of foam represents the rectum, the next the internal anal sphincter, the next the external anal sphincter.

Some videos feature a suturing simulator, where instead of foam the hands stitch together layers of silicone designed to simulate human muscle and skin and tissue. The thick flesh of the simulator looks and moves like raw filet mignon.

In the most realistic videos, the hands stitch together the deeply incised sides of a real beef tongue, through which beef tripe and chicken leg muscle have been tunneled to represent the anal mucosa and anal sphincter.

Most of the videos are silent, but a few feature instructors who warn about the dangers of misidentifying or improperly repairing OASIS, who speak clinically about fecal incontinence and fistulas. They are talking to medical students and residents. They are not thinking about me and my curiosity, my cold coffee in the early dark, pressing replay.

Almost all of the videos have comments turned off, but the ones that don't are full of replies from women whose stitches have burst or who didn't get the stitches they needed in the first place. They want to know if it's too late, will they always be in pain, how much does it cost.

LEAVE: PART III

Given my situation, I was happy with ten weeks of leave.

But at ten weeks, I am not recovered. At ten weeks, I am just beginning the months of weekly pelvic floor therapy appointments that it will take to break up the massive amounts of scar tissue inside my vaginal canal and return my bladder to where it belongs. At ten weeks, I still have an undiagnosed anal fissure that makes it impossible to sit comfortably and causes random stabbing pain throughout the day. At ten weeks, I am sleep-deprived and fumbling my way through learning how to pump, my engorged breasts demanding attention every two hours.

At ten weeks, I don't have a place to work because I work from home and the baby is too young for any of the local daycares. We can't afford a nanny, but we can (barely) afford a nanny share, so we pool our resources with another family in the neighborhood. The other mother, though, has more leave than I do, so we are on our own for now, and the nanny and the baby need the apartment. I sign up for a service that gives me day passes to coworking spaces. The service is cheaper than a regular coworking membership, but the catch is that you can only go to the same place twice in a month. Every day I pack my computer, my pump, and bags and ice packs for the milk and take the subway or the bus (or both, with a transfer) to one of the ten closest spaces, some of which are a 45-minute commute each way.

Only one of these spaces has what is euphemistically called a "mother's room" and the days I am there feel luxurious compared to the days I spend pumping in bathroom stalls or Starbucks bathrooms or in the back-seats of Lyfts or, once, desperately, because the train was stalled and I was starting to leak, on the subway. My work days are already cut short by the commute because we can't afford more than eight hours of childcare, so the additional time spent pumping between client calls stresses me out, and the stress affects my milk supply and makes the pumping sessions longer. Some days it takes me 20 minutes to get two ounces, so I add extra sessions after work and in the middle of the night to make sure the baby has enough for the next day.

At ten weeks, I am not ready to return to work, but I do. I am intellectually and emotionally absent during meetings. I get the bare minimum done on some of my projects. Others do not get done. This is not a way I have ever worked before and I am not okay with it, but it's all I can manage. I consider leaving the job altogether. We need the paycheck and the health insurance, but what my body needs is rest, and without it, my recovery stretches longer and longer.

GOOD BABIES

The woman who taught our birth class told us not to use the term "good baby." The idea of some babies being good babies means that others are bad babies. "All babies are good babies," she said.

Still, I find myself telling people that we have a good baby. People ask if he is sleeping and I insist that yes, he is sleeping beautifully. He took to feeding, he barely cries. An easy baby.

"He's not," Daniel says when we are alone. "You say that, but he's not."

Daniel is right. The baby, like most babies, wakes up multiple times a night and is difficult to put back down. The baby, like most babies, is especially cranky for one to two hours every evening. He is not a colicky baby and he is not sick, but taking care of him is challenging in the way that taking care of any baby is challenging.

I keep insisting I have an easy baby because I have used this tactic all my life: if I do not admit how hard things are, they won't be hard. I have long believed in the power of language to shape our experience. What we call things matters. And yet, with each passing month, "easy" feels more like an unstable facade I have built around my real house, one that all the neighbors can see through anyway.

I don't want to remember my baby's early years this way: the first year brimming with pain that flowed into the second, a pandemic, and the third, more pandemic. I have the power to tell a happy story. I am able, technically, to craft a narrative about obstacles overcome. But to do so would be inauthentic to the life lived in these years, a life which has been mostly hard with bright, soft spots.

Sometimes I wonder—is the person I am post-injury worse than who I was before? Did I waste this opportunity to grow in compassion, to better understand the pain of others, by allowing myself to wallow too long in self-pity and regret?

But the sole purpose of pain is not to make us better people, because there is no sole purpose of pain. We all do with it what we will, and sometimes all we can do is get through.

FISSURE

The obstetrician says the tear is healing nicely, but I still experience constant shooting pain, and I still fear going to the bathroom. After most bowel movements, I have to lie down and recover for thirty to sixty minutes, until the area feels less exposed and inflamed. I must still be extremely careful about what I eat; even yellow mustard is too spicy and will make my bathroom trips worse. I still have hemorrhoids the size of marbles, but I know those are fairly normal. There is a different pain, a not-normal pain, I feel I must insist; this doctor's appointment, for which I had to take time off work when I am already so behind, feels like a last chance to be heard.

"The pain," I say, "is in my anus," and my doctor seems visibly uncomfortable.

"Your anus?" she repeats.

Have I used the wrong clinical term? Am I, after all this, a stranger to my own body?

"My anus," I say. But the doctor assures me that everything is fine.

I insist it is not, and the doctor acknowledges that this is not her area of expertise. She suggests that I see a gastroenterologist.

The gastroenterologist is an empathetic listener. He himself has celiac disease, and so he knows about difficult bathroom trips. He does a careful physical exam and diagnoses an anal fissure, a tear in the mucosa that lines the anus.

Relief, just hearing the word fissure. Yes! I have been split in two. Giving birth caused a physical fracture in my life. I am now forced daily to examine the fault line.

I have questions. Is it related to the tearing from the birth, or is this something different? Was the grade of my tear correctly diagnosed?

The gastroenterologist, since he is only seeing me now, can't say, but he is optimistic that the fissure can be treated and healed in a matter of months. Months, I think. It has already been months.

He orders a medication from a compounding pharmacy to be delivered to my apartment along with a bag of one hundred latex finger cots, which look like miniature condoms. Every night for the next ten weeks, I roll one over my index finger and carefully apply the medication. Every night, I cry, sometimes because it is painful and sometimes because the pain has become an echo I worry I will always hear.

AN ABRIDGED SEARCH HISTORY, PART III

what is a fever baby
can you mix breast milk from different days
sex after third degree tear
baby making gasping sucking noise
how to treat bladder prolapse
how often should a baby eat 16 weeks
pelvic organ prolapse will sex make it worse
one breast makes more milk than other
how often to pump during workday
4 months postpartum still can't have sex
anal fissure when will i recover

VAGINAL ATROPHY

Vaginal intercourse is impossible; everything feels too tight, and upon the slightest entry, I feel as if the skin inside my vagina is being flayed.

The pelvic floor therapist tells me it's partially my injury—the scar tissue is still fresh and inflamed—and partially vaginal atrophy, a horrific term for the thinning, drying, and inflammation of the vaginal walls that can be caused by a drop in estrogen. It usually happens during menopause but can also happen to breastfeeding women. I message my doctor about it and she prescribes an estrogen cream, but I am scared off by the many all-caps warnings about cancer that come with the prescription and never use it.

The pelvic floor therapist suggests vaginal dilators, a set of plastic bullet-shaped implements that are inserted in the vaginal cavity to stretch the walls. The idea is to begin with the smallest dilator in the set and work your way up to the largest.

I recall hearing once that Virginia Woolf had vaginismus, and though now I can find no record or real evidence of this, the possibility of it casts new light on her writing about illness. I wonder about her private pain. We know about the emotional turmoil, we know about the bouts of flu. But was there pain she felt she could not entirely describe, even to Leonard, even to Vanessa, even to her doctors—even to Vita? I return to this passage from *The Waves:*

> But for pain words are lacking. There should be cries, cracks, fissures, whiteness passing over chintz covers, interference with the sense of time, of space; the sense also of extreme fixity in passing objects; and sounds very remote and then very close; flesh being gashed and blood spurting, a joint suddenly twisted—beneath all of which appears something very important, yet remote, to be just held in solitude.

ANOTHER VISITATION

Heather tells me that her dad has been very sick and can no longer breathe.

Heather is not afraid of death. After her step-dad died when she was sixteen, she tells me, he began to send her signs from the afterlife.

I love listening to Heather talk about her encounters with the supernatural because it makes me feel like I could believe in something again. She's gotten into psychedelics and recently spent an evening having an out-of-body experience in Janis Joplin's old room at the Chelsea Hotel doing a drug she calls "the medicine," which comes from the venom of a toad. According to Heather, the medicine rewires one's brain, eases anxiety and depression, opens a person's eyes to the ways in which we are connected.

Her step-dad's messages, Heather tells me, always come through songs. Sometimes it's "Here Comes the Sun," sometimes "Layla," sometimes "Wonderful Tonight." He spoke to her after her brother died of cancer a couple of years ago, and it was all three songs in a row, sung by a busker in a town square in Croatia. She closes her eyes as she describes how her body reacted to this communication from beyond, and I can see that she is preparing for her dad's death. She is readying herself for his visit.

OCCULT

I come across the term "occult anal sphincter injury," an injury of the anal sphincter that is either clinically undetectable or is missed immediately after delivery but is able to be diagnosed later using an endoanal ultrasound.

The medical literature suggests that more are missed than are truly undetectable. "Interestingly," one article notes, "repair of the internal anal sphincter is not described in standard obstetric textbooks." Another article, published in the year I got pregnant, says that "recent studies have noted that obstetrics and gynecology residents are poorly trained to identify and repair third and fourth degree lacerations."

The very existence of these occult injuries would seem to indicate that the rate of OASIS is underreported. There are more of us out there, I think.

I wonder about the other women, how long it took them to walk, how many of them are still in pain three months, six months, a year or more later. I wonder how many of them struggle with their symptoms in silence because they don't know what to call them, because their doctors have dismissed them, because they're too busy taking care of their kids to tend to an invisible injury.

PLOT

The baby babbles.

"Are you telling me a story?" I say.

He gurgles.

"How does the story begin?" I say. "What happens first? And then what happens? And then what?"

As if anything is linear.

My grandmother winds up in the hospital again, this time with a respiratory infection, but she is there long enough for a detox. This has happened before: a new team of doctors trying to coax her onto a different path. Maybe now will be the time that it works. I speak with her on the phone. She says she wants to go home.

WANTED

After my grandmother recovers, she and my mother get in a fight over something silly that is a cover for something deeper. They have gone through long periods of silence before, but this is the longest. It will stretch on for months and months and will only end when my Grandpa Duke is admitted to the hospital, where he will die.

My grandmother and my mother are alike in many ways: hurt, hard, stubborn. When one of them harms the other, they curl up like armadillos and roll into their separate corners. Until my sister came along, our family had carved no path to forgiveness. Our ancestors made no apologies. They doubled down on their wrongdoings.

"Nobody talks to me like that," my grandmother tells me over the phone, indignant, reliving what she claims my mother said, words my mother will dispute.

"You still love her," I say.

"Eh," my grandmother says. In her cruel dismissal, I hear the echo of her own mother, a woman who chose to walk away.

I often wonder how things would have been different for my grandmother, for my mother, for me, had my grandmother been a wanted baby.

I wanted my baby and having him is still so hard. I don't blame my great-grandmother for leaving, when she had so few choices in the first place, but I am sad for her, and for my grandmother, and for my mother, and for me.

LIVING

As the months go on, I stop providing updates to my friends. Who wants to hear that someone who was in pain is still in pain? Who wants to hear that someone who looks fine is still in pain? The story is supposed to be one of healing; what was torn should be made whole.

When I was pregnant, I asked my sister if she had experienced the horrible pregnancy hemorrhoids I was dealing with.

"Yes," she said. "And they never really went away."

"You have got to be shitting me," I wanted to say but did not say because I don't swear around my sister.

"They pop out during the day," she explained, "and every morning in the shower, I just pop them back in."

"Same," my mother said when I told her about my sister. I was nearly sick to my stomach.

Now I see how the days go by, though things are not as they should be. How we go on living.

DYING

The living body is dying. Cells die and are replaced by other cells. The mass of cells we lose each year through normal cell death is close to our entire body weight. Our regenerative capabilities slow with age. Before long, the shedding and relining of my uterus will cease for good. If I break a bone now, it will be more difficult for my skeletal muscle cells to regenerate. If I break a bone twenty years from now, even more so. Waiting for my body to heal all these months, I have never felt closer to death.

On the other hand, it is encouraging: we have the ability to completely remake ourselves. I am not made of the same stuff I was at 16, at 26. In some ways, I am stronger and braver.

The living body is dying, but the living body is also living, living with the baby who now pulls himself to stand, who calls her ma ma ma, who just saw the ocean for the first time.

PORTAL

Heather's dad dies. We are in her apartment, which smells of mugwort and is full of books about metaphysics, when she tells me about it, how she flew to Virginia not knowing how long he had and ended up staying several weeks. How she watched him struggle to breathe, move in and out of lucidity. How her step-mom switched out the oxygen tanks twice a day.

We have this conversation looking into each other's eyes in a mirror, because she is cutting my hair again. It is an intimate way to talk about death, her hands on my scalp.

She tells me she has decided to become a death doula. She's enrolled in an official training program, with a whole cohort of people preparing to usher their fellow humans across this final threshold.

She tells me what she already knows about death: the order in which the body shuts itself down during the natural death process. How the desire to eat diminishes, and with it the body's creation of waste. "A dying person can take days to fill a whole catheter bag, and the urine will be dark," she says. She tells me how the legs and feet swell from edema.

Then she tells me about the hallucinations, the visions.

How a person can be in the room yet not present at all. How the body returns to its most animal.

"It sounds like birth," I say.

"It's the same portal," Heather says. "We all come in through it, and we all go out."

THE MOM GENE

"You didn't get the mom gene," my mother tells me after observing me with the baby.

"That's not very nice," I say, trying to laugh off the sting.

"It's not a bad thing," she says. "I didn't get it either. We're not like your sister, happy to stay at home with the kids all day. This," she says, meaning the week we are spending with the baby because his daycare is closed for summer break, "is not what we would choose to do with our time."

She is not wrong about that.

CLASSIC RERUNS

When I was a kid, my mother helped my grandmother open a resale shop.

At the time, my grandmother was working the cash register at a busy truck stop off the interstate. My sister and I loved to visit her at work because she would give us a bagful of quarters for the claw machine, and if we made it through the whole bag without winning, she would open the machine using one of the many keys on her large metal ring and let us each pick out a toy anyway. This was another thing a grandmother was: someone who always had the key.

My mother felt that my grandmother deserved to be more in charge of her work and her time. She had worked so hard, for so long, for other people. The way my mother saw it, the resale shop was a way out.

She helped my grandmother find a storefront to rent. They acquired steel clothing racks and set up mirrors in curtained dressing rooms. My mother came up with a clever name and stenciled a sign to hang outside the shop: Classic Reruns.

At first, my grandmother was enthusiastic. She loved going to garage sales, and this was like one never-ending garage sale. She enjoyed talking to the people who came in to browse or sell their things on consignment. She ended up buying many of the items herself, and they piled up in her basement. She often gave things away for free. She wasn't a very shrewd shop owner.

And she quickly grew bored. There weren't enough customers at the resale shop, and she was often alone for hours at a time. At the truck stop, the lines were always long and the shifts flew by. Plus, she didn't get the same satisfaction from working for herself; she liked accumulating hours and cashing them out in the form of a regular paycheck.

She got a job at a gas station in the next town over and left my Grandpa Duke to run the shop, which he did for many years. Owning a business, it turned out, was my mother's dream.

AMERICA

I run into a neighbor, a woman who is new to this country. She is standing on our street, observing a group of cop cars at the entrance of the building next door to mine, lights on, no sirens. It is 3 o'clock on a Friday afternoon. Shots have been fired into an apartment from the street, my neighbor tells me.

She is distressed, but not just about that. She tells me of her difficulty finding a gynecologist in New York. She is trying to navigate the American insurance system, but each time she thinks she has found a doctor who takes her plan, the appointment falls through. Now, an appointment that has been on the books for a month has just been canceled at the last minute because, according to the administrator who called, "the doctor decided not to come in today."

My neighbor is frustrated and tells me she really needs to see someone. Her son is three, but she is still dealing with symptoms from the birth.

We talk around it for a while; we don't know each other well. Eventually, we realize we had the same injury, mine after a quick birth, hers following a long and difficult one, her son's shoulder stuck in the birth canal.

"For me it was the anal tear that was the killer," I say as two cops walk by. My neighbor nods. More cop cars arrive, driving the wrong way up our one-way street.

She describes the pain of being immediately separated from her newborn and is surprised to hear that I was not. Any tear of the third degree and above and you go straight to the OR, where she is from.

I consider whether or not I would have been better off that way. There is no way to know, but at least I got to hold and feed my baby as the stitches went in. And here she is, asking me the name of my pelvic floor therapist, neither of us completely healed.

DO-OVER

Another neighbor, a woman who experienced preterm labor and an emergency C-section with her first child, gets pregnant again and vows to have a home birth this time. The way she talks about it, it sounds like she wants vindication, or to recover something that she lost in the hospital. I get it.

When the baby is nearly two, I miss a period. On a hot, humid day, I walk to the pharmacy on the corner to get a test and a family-size bottle of ibuprofen. The woman working the counter winks at me.

Over the next two weeks, I pee on six sticks. Every test is negative, and yet I fail to bleed.

I imagine getting another chance, like my neighbor. Doing a home birth, allowing the baby to come when it wants to come. Assembling a team of birth workers I trust. Not going anywhere near the hospital.

Of course, I could still wind up there. I could need an emergency C-section, I could hemorrhage. But I allow myself to envision a second birth that goes well, that does not result in months of pain.

"I could have a do-over," I say.

"That's not a good reason to have a child," my therapist says.

I google "chances of a third or fourth degree tear on second birth" and find that a greater percentage of those who have experienced this degree of tearing opt for elective C-sections the second time around. For those who don't, the chances of tearing in the same way again are quadrupled.

I wait, despairing. Finally, after many weeks, I bleed.

BIRTH STORIES, PART III

I am actually certain that I do not want another baby. Partially, it comes down to money.

We spent a large chunk of our savings to have a baby, and we are some of the privileged ones; while it was a stretch to spend it—and while it was infuriating to think about the $12,000 a year we were already paying in premiums just to have health insurance, only to find that our health insurance didn't fully cover birth—we had the money at the end of the day. There are families who fall into serious debt after childbirth.

Just like every birth has a birth story, every birth story in this country has a financial breakdown. This is ours.

At the time I gave birth, New York's Paid Family Leave covered 10 weeks of leave at 60% of one's pay, unless that pay was above the average salary in New York State (at the time, a little under $47,000 a year), in which case the weekly payments were capped at 60% of the average. This payment was taxed, and after taxes, I was just glad that the amount covered the healthcare premiums I still owed while I was on leave from work. Over half of the money we got from Paid Family Leave went straight to the health insurance company.

Given this, I expected that our birth would be fully covered and was surprised when the bills began to arrive. The hospital charged over $30,000 for the birth, $18,000 of which was covered by our health insurance. The explanation of benefits informed me that the remaining $12,000 was up to us to cover. Around $9,000 of it was for 36 hours of "room and board" at the hospital following the birth—a shared room for a night and a half.

"What about our deductible? What about out-of-pocket maximums?" I asked when I called the insurance company, trying to understand. But the charges had been split cleverly between me and the baby—apparently newborns must pay their own "room and board"—because we each had an individual deductible to meet, and some charges didn't count toward our deductible or out-of-pocket maximums because they weren't covered services to begin with.

What we owed was broken up into several bills, some from the doctor's office, some from the hospital, and some from some entity that I was informed was not the hospital but related to the hospital. For the largest invoice, the hospital offered to set us up on an interest-free payment plan. A few hundred dollars a month to slowly whittle away our debt over time.

I made many calls, some to the insurance company but most to the hospital because the baby had been entered into their system with both the wrong name and the wrong address, which made sorting out the invoices even more confusing. During one of these calls, I joked to the woman on the phone that I was hoping the billing mix-up might mean the charges for the baby were forgiven. She laughed. Then she said she needed to talk to her supervisor and that someone would call me back. No one ever called me back, but a $3,000 charge was erased from our online account. I was shocked and grateful but also terrified that it might just be another mistake, so I never called again.

My company was self-funding its medical plan that year, and part of that arrangement involved covering a percentage of out-of-pocket employee costs once they passed the $2,500 mark. As a result, a portion of what we spent on covered services was reimbursed to us at the end of the year, one lump-sum deposit into our bank account, which, though I still felt the insurance plan should have covered more of the costs, was a huge help.

At the end of the day, we spent around $7,000 on the birth and the prenatal appointments leading up to it. At the same time, we paid entirely out of pocket for my first round of pelvic floor therapy, which was not covered at all and amounted to around $2,000.

I hate that it can cost so much to have a baby in this country, and that the price you pay depends on how the birth goes, what the hospital bills, and how the insurance company processes the claims, making it impossible to plan for those costs ahead of time.

I hate that I felt forced to return to work before I was ready in order to keep an expensive health insurance plan that didn't even cover the physical therapy I needed.

I hate that the childcare that allowed me to return to work was somehow both more expensive than we could afford and also undervalued in terms of the labor it actually required.

And so my body tells me that I do not want another child, and my mind and my heart agree.

WORKING MOMS

Over the phone, I ask my mother again how she felt about her mother working. "I always got the impression that you were proud of her for being a working mother at a time when not many were," I say.

"I'm proud of her work ethic," my mother clarifies. "But she was needed at home. It was hard on us."

"Do you think she would have been happy if she'd been a stay-at-home mom?" I ask. We both know my grandmother would have been miserable. I want my mother to acknowledge the thing she and I and my grandmother share, the inability to completely shed our other identities in order to take on the mantle of mother. I don't see this as a bad thing.

"No, she wouldn't have, because she always had to have her own money. It was a control thing. She grew up with no money, and she wanted enough that she could leave if she needed to. She didn't want to be stuck."

"Fair enough," I say.

"And maybe there was a little guilt. Grandpa Duke took in three kids, so maybe she felt like she needed to help. But he had a good job. She could have stayed home."

"Do you wish she had stayed home?"

"Yes."

"Do you wish you had stayed home?"

"No."

"How is it different?"

"I went to college. I had career aspirations. Plus, I didn't want to stay home all day. I didn't think that would be good for me or for you guys, and when I say you didn't get the mom gene, that's what I mean. I wasn't being critical of you."

"For the record, I don't wish you had stayed home," I say. "But I also get the sense that Grandma is the same way. Staying at home would have driven her completely crazy."

"It wasn't just the fact that she worked, but the shift that she chose to work, two to eleven. She says three to eleven, but she always left at two, and she didn't get home til midnight. She was still sleeping when we left for school. We were left to our own devices. I never would have put the onus on you to raise your siblings or run a household."

It's clear that thinking about this is painful for my mother, and she is far from seeing her experience as similar to her own mother's. She won't even allow that wanting to earn one's own money, to not be stuck relying on a man, might qualify as a career aspiration. But I can see it, this thing she wants to call a gene, coming down from my great-grandmother and maybe her mother before her, the one who was brave enough to start over in a new country: a lineage of women who wanted something different than what was offered to them.

THE WOUNDED HEALER

A mother is a hole that gets bigger and bigger as we throw things in—our love, our expectations, our disappointments, our shame. And then the hole starts to close up, until there is nothing left but a seam. One long suture. A scar.

"A mother is a wound," I find myself saying to people I don't even know very well.

When I say wound, I mean like Chiron, the minor planet. Named for the centaur in Greek mythology who had the power to heal others but could not heal himself, Chiron is referred to by astrologers as the wounded healer, and its placement in one's birth chart is said to reveal the wound that is one's life's work. Mine is in Gemini, in the seventh house of relationships, yet another reminder of my need for an other.

This is the material I have to work with if I want healing. If I engage with the teachings of this wound, I may even become a healer myself.

STITCHED, PART III

At my first postpartum annual GYN appointment, when the baby is a year old, I tell the doctor that my recovery is going okay, but that I used to run half-marathons and now I can't even run a mile. Even a slow jog for a minute or two causes a bulging pressure on my pelvic floor.

"I can't run a mile, and I haven't even had a baby," she says.

It is only the following year, when the baby is two, that my doctor seems more empathetic. She has a friend who recently had a third-degree tear, she tells me, a woman who is a pilates teacher and understands the pelvic floor. Even this woman—and here I wonder if she previously thought my injury was my fault, for not understanding my pelvic floor—could not avoid a long and painful recovery, and this personal experience seems to have shifted something in my doctor. "What you went through was difficult," she says, and this plain statement brings me to tears.

My doctor is relatively young; she was only six years out of medical school when my baby was born. If she was delivering babies that entire time at the rate of the national average, she might have delivered about 600. Add to that maybe 100 during her medical residency. It is possible that she only dealt with a handful of OASIS before encountering mine. I remember how proud she was of the way her stitches were healing in each of my follow-up appointments. It was the pride of someone who didn't get many chances to practice.

Initially, I assumed my doctor knew how bad my recovery was while it was happening but didn't say it for fear of scaring me or pushing me over the edge. Now, I think it's possible that she truly didn't get it until she saw her friend go through it.

BOTH

Over time, the constant pain will be reduced to flare-ups, but the flare-ups will persist for three more years until the gastroenterologist finally makes a referral to a colorectal surgeon. The colorectal surgeon will use an anoscope and what appears to be a headlamp to look inside me and will diagnose a rectocele, a prolapse of the rectum into the back wall of the vagina. No running, no jumping, no lifting, no cycling, no squats, she will say. She will send me back to pelvic floor therapy.

Months of pelvic floor therapy is something I won't have the time for, but I will find the time, along with the thousands more dollars it will cost. The pelvic floor therapist will tell me that she often sees this type of prolapse in the years after an extensive tear; the heaviness and tightness of the stitching can pull the rectum forward over time, she will say. And then she will put her healing hands inside me.

I still don't know whether my postpartum experience is extraordinary or banal. It's possible that, like life itself, like death, it is both.

A BIG HOUSE

Heather begins working on a documentary film series about the different ways to die.

"Most people don't want to die in the hospital," she says. We are back in her apartment, her hands in my hair. "Yet so many of us do, because we're not aware of the alternatives. Dying is something that every single one of us is going to experience. We want it to be with people who love us and care for us."

Heather describes to me her ideal death. She wants to rent a big house and invite all her friends to hang out.

I think of my pain after the birth, how I barely registered what was happening around me, how I was forced to dissociate from my body. I can't imagine, in that state, that it would be pleasurable to hang out in a big house with all my friends. I can't imagine, in that state, even transporting my body to a big house. The ability to achieve the ideal death, I think, depends on the way in which one's body dies, which is something most of us don't control. In this way, death is like birth. It is common for people to laugh at the naïveté of their birth plan after the fact.

I say none of this, because it is cynical. I still think there is value in making a birth plan. I'm still glad I made a birth playlist, even if my song choices seem ludicrously optimistic now. "A big house," I say. "It sounds lovely."

BIRTH: A PLAYLIST

Get Me Away From Here, I'm Dying
Can't Go Back Now
Here Comes My Baby
Don't Stop Me Now
Hips Don't Lie
Never Going Back Again
Nothing's Gonna Stop Us Now
Bring It On Home to Me
Hold You in My Arms
Fruits Of My Labor
The Obvious Child
Here at the Right Time
Naked as We Came
Heartbeats
Baby, Baby
Mother and Child Reunion
Two of Us
Welcome Home, Son

LEAVING

The baby has seen many sides of me. The baby has seen me with other people, performing. The baby has watched me get lost in my head and forget him. The baby learned early that there are ways we are when we're alone.

Now the baby is a toddler. Now the toddler goes to daycare and spends his days drumming on bongos, tracing his hand to make a paper turkey, planting beans in plastic bags with moist paper towels to learn how they sprout. Now the toddler doesn't want to be told what to do, says, "No!" Says, "I do it my own self."

It's strange to think of him going all these places without me, places I have never been. Each morning, he leaves me to go make his own days. One day, there will be a larger leaving, perhaps more than one. What the leave he takes will look like is impossible to know.

THE MOTHER

When the baby is no longer a baby but a small child, my mother will be diagnosed with breast cancer. While she is receiving radiation treatments in another state, my grandmother will go into hospice.

"You are my surrogate," my mother, tearful, will say to me over the phone. "Don't leave her alone." She begs the doctors to double up her radiation treatments, two per day, so that she can go home to her mother. Finally, they will agree, but she will miss the death by one day.

During my grandmother's rally—those mysterious hours just before a dying person's body really begins to shut down, when it seems they might be improving, might not be dying after all, and they experience a brief burst of lucidity—I will sit on the edge of her bed and rub her back. It will be the only time during her hospice stay when we are alone, all the uncles and cousins having left for the day. I will ask her if she is afraid.

"No," she will say. But then she will add, "I'm afraid of the pain."

I will make no promises about pain.

"She has to be the mother now," my grandmother will

tell me. “I can’t be the mother.”

“Who? My mom?”

“Yeah. She has to be the mother.”

I will jot down the other things she says so that I don’t forget. “Family is the most important thing to me.” “I can only be who I am.” She will tell me she is embarrassed about the way her hair looks. “I was supposed to get it done the day I went to the hospital.”

By the next day, she will be unable to talk and we will sit listening to the loud, rhythmic sucking of the oxygen machine. The hospice nurses will administer a steady course of morphine and benzodiazepines to keep her comfortable, but it will still look and sound painful.

“You’ve been through this before,” I will whisper to her. “This is your longest labor.”

After two days of the final stage of dying, I will call my mother. “She can’t speak, but I think she needs to hear your voice.” I will hold the phone up to my grandmother’s ear so my mother can talk to her. An hour later, my grandmother will let go.

IN THE CARDS

Rummaging through a drawer, I find the set of cards I made myself before the birth. I remember the night I made them, 38 weeks pregnant and unable to sleep. The heat, the heartburn, the Fourth of July fireworks lighting up the neighborhood. I sat cross-legged on the couch, cutting up thick brown kraft paper and writing mantras as they came into my head.

Some I'd seen on social media:

Every contraction brings me closer to my baby.
My baby knows how to be born.
My baby and I are working together.

Most were phrases I'd used when running:

I own this hill.
I'm doing the damn thing.
I can do anything for 60 seconds.
I am on no one's schedule but my own.

I strung the cards together and tucked them in my hospital bag, where they remained for a couple of months, until I finally gathered the energy to finish unpacking and banished them to the back of my sock drawer. In the aftermath of the birth, each mantra felt like a fresh indictment of my failures.

I trust my body?
My birth will go exactly as it should?

Now, I can see the cards for what they are: a best attempt to prepare for the unknown, and an act of care. One of the cards rings truer than the rest:

Everything changes.

Now, I am a mother, one who is still able to talk to her own mother and grandmother. One day, I will be something else.

ACKNOWLEDGEMENTS

Thank you to Michael Wheaton for bringing *Leave* into the world. When you said, "It pretends to be a book about birth, but it's really a book about death," I knew I had found the right home. Thanks to the whole Autofocus team, especially Amy Wheaton for illustrating the book cover of my dreams.

To my agent, Ashley Lopez, thank you for believing in my work all these years. I love being part of the family you're building.

Thank you to the members of my writing groups, past and present, including Sarah Kunstler, Brian Zimbler, Paul Perkus, Aron Mesh, Martin Anderson, Alice Kaltman, Chris Gonzalez, Melanie Faranello, Jenny Halper, Tony Tulathimutte and my CRIT cohort, Julián Delgado Lopera and my Tin House workshop, Chelsea Hodson and the whole Morning Writing Club, Jami Attenberg and everyone who keeps coming back for more 1000 Words of Summer, and especially to Rachel León and Maureen Langloss for reading the first draft of *Leave* and giving me the confidence to start calling it a book.

Sara Lippmann, meeting you changed the course of my life. You showed me how to be a writer in this world. You were the first to encourage me to submit my work. The way you talk about fiction is magical. Thank you for being my mentor and my friend and for being so gracious when my baby spit up all over you at that word west reading in 2019. This book would not exist without you.

For your kind and generous words in support of *Leave*, thank you to Lexi Kent-Monning, Sue Rainsford, Carley Moore, Lindsay Hunter, Elisa Albert, and Jiordan Castle. Thank you to Erin Slaughter for your thoughtful notes.

Thank you to the people who lived these days with me: Leslie Brand, Anna Chapin, Bailey Edgell, Sofia Frank, Megan Harrington, Sarah Schillaci, Alison Lewis, Cindy Choung, Boris Rasin, Elyse Benedicto, Ashley Frank Clausen, Sarah Mannone, and Fionnuala Barrett.

Matt and Charlene Warner, thank you for your friendship and for doing whatever it took to rescue our dog on the night of the birth.

Natasha Sardesai-Grant, there is no one with whom I'd rather share a labor and delivery nurse. Thank you for all the advice, for checking on me so often in those postpartum weeks and months, and for coming to sit with me that day when my sister had gone home and my mom had not yet arrived. You helped me feel less alone.

Heather Hogan, you have taught me so much about life and death. I love to see the world through your eyes, and I'm so glad the universe brought me to your chair.

Missy Middleton, you believed in me before I believed in myself. You may not have been my teacher, but you have been my teacher.

Sarah Saffian, you saw me through it all. Thank you.

Thank you, Raychel Franzen, for helping me hold the baby in until we got to the hospital. Thank you, Shani Fried and Michele McGurk, for the pelvic floor physical therapy and the hope. Thank you, Bernice Stewart and Pauline Talloch, for caring for our baby (and, by extension, our family) with such fierce love.

I truly won the in-law lottery; thank you to Albert Mazzone, David Mazzone, Hannah Schofield, and especially to Dawn Mazzone for your love and care.

To my dad, thank you for always accepting me.

To my sister, thank you for being there, for your grace, and for your intentionality. It is a gift to watch you mother.

To my mom, thank you for flying out a second time; you always seem to know when I need you but don't want to ask for help. One of the best things about becoming a parent is how it's deepened my relationship with you. Another is witnessing your love for my kid.

Thank you, Daniel, for handling every nighttime feeding, changing every diaper, administering every bath, and taking on a ton of extra household labor while I recovered. You are my first reader, my partner in all things, and an amazing dad. We are so lucky to have you.

Finally, thank you, Gus, for being you.

ABOUT THE AUTHOR

Shayne Terry's work has appeared in *American Chordata, Catapult, Chicago Review of Books, CRAFT, Electric Literature, TriQuarterly, Vol. 1 Brooklyn,* and elsewhere. She has been selected for workshops and residencies at Bread Loaf, Tin House, and the Vermont Studio Center.

Born and raised in northern Illinois, Shayne received an M.A. in Literature from University College Dublin and lives in Brooklyn.

shayneterry.com

— also from Autofocus Books —

Duplex — Mike Nagel

XO — Sara Rauch

Until It Feels Right — Emily Costa

Cleave — Holly Pelesky

Nextdoor in Colonialtown — Ryan Rivas

Too Much Tongue — Adrienne Marie Barrios & Leigh Chadwick

Picture Window — Danny Caine

the nature machine! — Tyler Gillespie

A Kind of In-Between — Aaron Burch

How to Write a Novel: An Anthology of 20 Craft Essays About Writing, None of Which Ever Mention Writing — ed. Aaron Burch

Hiraeth — Mistie R. Watkins

That Spell — Tate N. Oquendo

My Modest Blindness — Russell Brakefield

A Calendar Is A Snakeskin — Kristine Langley Mahler

Culdesac — Mike Nagel

Razed by TV Sets — Jason McCall

In the Away Time — Kristen E. Nelson

The Body Is A Temporary Gathering Place — Andrew Bertaina

Daughterhood — Emily Adrian

A Healthy Interest in the Lives of Others — Teresa Carmody

Yes I Am Human I Know You Were Wondering — Erin Dorney